Anesthesia Management for Electroconvulsive Therapy

Shigeru Saito
Editor

Anesthesia Management for Electroconvulsive Therapy

Practical Techniques and Physiological Background

Springer

Editor
Shigeru Saito
Department of Anesthesiology
Gunma University Graduate School of Medicine
Maebashi
Japan

ISBN 978-4-431-56682-3 ISBN 978-4-431-55717-3 (eBook)
DOI 10.1007/978-4-431-55717-3

Softcover reprint of the hardcover 1st edition 2016

Printed on acid-free paper

This Springer imprint is published by Springer Nature
The registered company is Springer Japan KK

Preface

Electroconvulsive therapy (ECT) was introduced in clinical practice based on the finding that psychiatric symptoms are improved after a seizure in a patient suffering from both schizophrenia and epilepsy. In spite of the great effort expended, the underlying mechanism has not been fully elucidated. ECT therapy has undergone several decades of criticism, accusations of inappropriate use, legal restrictions, and public protest. However, recent controlled studies have demonstrated clinical benefits of this therapy and many efforts have been made to reduce the special risks in ECT. Specifically, the introduction of general anesthesia using intravenous anesthetics and a muscle relaxant greatly reduced physical risks relating the muscular convulsive movement during the therapy. Currently, ECT for drug therapy-resistant depression and some other psychiatric disorders is widely accepted as a safe and effective therapy. Use of ECT for several psychiatric conditions is expanding, and the number of patients receiving ECT is increasing.

Although the basic mechanism of the clinical effects of ECT has not been clarified, several authorized medical societies, including the Royal College of Psychiatrists in the United Kingdom and the American Psychiatric Association, have published guidelines and audit-reports to promote the safe and effective use of ECT and to prevent its misuse. According to such guidelines, this therapy is applied under general anesthesia in most advanced countries. Apparently, this approach is more safe and effective compared to the original method without anesthesia. The most recent version of the guideline by the American Psychiatric Association clearly stated that anesthesia for ECT should be administered by a specially trained anesthesiologist, and that the anesthesiologists should have overall responsibility, not only for anesthesia itself but also for cardiopulmonary management and emergency care.

Under these circumstances, anesthesiologists who administer anesthesia for ECT should have sufficient knowledge regarding the physiologically and pharmacologically unique effects of ECT. However, the number of descriptions regarding the anesthesia management for ECT is limited, and most such descriptions are relatively short review articles. A handy practical guidebook is considered to be attractive for young doctors and co-medical staffs working on this therapy. This ECT anesthesia guidebook is prepared to respond to such requests from clinicians.

Seven experts in this field earnestly reviewed recent clinical and basic literature regarding ECT anesthesia and described most updated knowledge in plain language. As editor, I believe that anesthesiologists, psychiatrists, and the other medical staff working on ECT can master ECT anesthesia by reading this guidebook and by applying the techniques to their clinical cases.

Maebashi, Japan Shigeru Saito

Contents

Pre-procedural Assessments and Considerations

1

Shigeki Yamaguchi and Toshifumi Takasusuki

Abstract

Electric stimulus and seizure during the electroconvulsive therapy (ECT) make patients various impacts so that it is recommended to perform ECT under general anesthesia (modified ECT: mECT). To optimize the anesthetic management of patients under mECT, it is important to understand the physiologic responses to the electrical stimulus, even though under general anesthesia. And also, the early assessment of patient's physical condition is required, since there may be some physical problems because of psychiatric disorders, medications and others in patients required for mECT. Therefore, pre-procedure assessment, including inquiry, check of medications and usual examinations, is also important and required as normal general anesthesia. If needed, special examinations and special monitor during anesthesia should be ordered. In this chapter, some points for pre-procedure assessments and conditions for mECT were described.

Keywords

Depression • Schizophrenia • Antidepressant • Antipsychotic • QT prolongation

1.1 Introduction

Electroconvulsive therapy (ECT) is a useful therapy for many psychiatric disorders, and the number of indications for which it is used is expanding (Table 1.1) [1–3]. Initially, ECT was performed without any anesthesia, resulting in serious problems such as fractures, tooth damage, and cardiovascular events, among others.

S. Yamaguchi (✉) • T. Takasusuki
Department of Anesthesiology, School of Medicine, Dokkyo Medical University, 880 Kitakobayashi, Mibu, Tochigi 321-0293, Japan
e-mail: shigeki@dokkyomed.ac.jp

S. Saito (ed.), *Anesthesia Management for Electroconvulsive Therapy*,
DOI 10.1007/978-4-431-55717-3_1

Table 1.1 Psychiatric diagnoses for which mECT has been claimed to be effective

1.	Major depression, single or recurrent episode
2.	Bipolar major depression, depressed or mixed type
3.	Bipolar disorder, mania or mixed type
4.	Schizophrenia
	Catatonia
	Schizophreniform or schizoaffective disorder
5.	Atypical psychosis
6.	Other conditions
	Organic delusional disorder
	Organic mood disorder
	Acute psychotic disorder
	Obsessive-compulsive disorder
	Dysthymia
7.	Miscellaneous conditions
	Parkinson's disease
	Neuroleptic malignant syndrome
	Secondary catatonia
	Lethal catatonia

As a result, it is now common to perform ECT while the patient is under general anesthetic [4].

The spread of modified ECT (mECT) has increased the number of psychiatric patients undergoing ECT. Currently, more mECT is performed than coronary artery bypass or appendectomy in the USA [2]. Furthermore, meta-analysis data have indicated that mECT may be more effective than antidepressants [5, 6].

Although electric stimuli and seizures affect patients in a variety of ways, anesthetic management for mECT may not have been given sufficiently serious consideration. However, anesthetic management of mECT must be considered in the same way as other cases undergoing general anesthesia, because hypnotics and muscle relaxants are required. Particular attention must also be paid to patients requiring mECT, as their conditions can be complicated and high risk.

Therefore, mECT must involve anesthesiologists who specialize in anesthetic management. Guidelines by the American Psychiatric Association state that collaboration with trained anesthesiologists can make mECT safer [6]. This chapter describes points to note regarding pre-procedure assessments and specific conditions in mECT.

1.2 Indications and Contraindications for mECT [7]

mECT is a useful therapy for many psychiatric and other disorders, especially drug-resistant conditions (Table 1.2). Table 1.3 lists symptoms that are responsive to ECT, indicating the wide variety of conditions for which mECT can be useful.

Table 1.2 Criteria for primary use and mECT

Situations in which ECT should be considered prior to a trial of psychotropic agents include the following:	
1.	Where a need for rapid, definitive recovery exists on either medical or psychiatric grounds
2.	When the risks of other treatments outweigh the risks of ECT
3.	When a history of poor drug response and/or good ECT response exists in previous episodes of the illness
4.	Patient preference

Table 1.3 Symptoms responsive to mECT

1.	Symptoms associated with depression: suicidal ideation, depressed mood, delusions of guilt, hypochondriasis
2.	Symptoms associated with other functional psychoses: depression, stupor, psychomotor excitement, delusions or illusions, anxiety, or agitation
3.	Secondary depression or confusion associated with various physical diseases
4.	Muscular rigidity associated with parkinsonism or neuroleptic malignant syndrome

On the other hand, mECT is contraindicated in some conditions. For instance, intracranial hypertension is an absolute contraindication; relative contraindications include intracranial lesion, cerebral aneurysm, recent myocardial infarction, angina pectoris, heart failure, untreated glaucoma, severe fractures, thrombophlebitis, pregnancy, and retinal detachment, among others.

1.3 Physiologic Responses to mECT [4, 8–12]

To optimize the management of anesthesia in patients undergoing mECT, an understanding of the physiologic responses to electrical stimulus is important. An electrical current applied to the brain via transcutaneous electrodes induces a systemic tonic-clonic seizure, usually comprising a tonic phase lasting 10–15 s and a tonic phase for 30–60 s.

During the tonic phase, the parasympathetic nervous system is activated, resulting in bradycardia and hypotension. Immediately afterwards, the clonic phase activates the sympathetic nervous system, resulting in tachycardia and hypertension. Although changes that appear similar to myocardial ischemia on electrocardiogram occur immediately after electrical stimulus, cardiac enzyme levels usually do not increase.

Electrical stimulus and subsequent seizure increase both cerebral blood flow and cerebral metabolism, leading to intracranial hypertension. Intraocular pressure and gastric pressure also increase after mECT.

1.4 Assessment of Patients before mECT [4, 13, 14]

The pre-procedure examination is as important and necessary as for general anesthesia in healthy subjects. Since patients requiring mECT may also have physical problems, early assessment of their physical condition is necessary. Special examinations may be necessary.

1.4.1 Inquiry

Certain details, such as complications, medical history, anesthetic history, and medication lists, among others, must be carefully checked. Since communication with patients requiring mECT can be difficult, it may be necessary to ask the patient's family and attending physicians.

1.4.2 Pre-procedure Examination (Table 1.4)

A regular examination should be conducted and evaluated in the same way as for any normal general anesthesia. Abdominal X-ray is required because bowel dysfunction may occur in some patients. The QT interval must be carefully checked via electrocardiogram because many patients requiring mECT may exhibit QT interval prolongation. Brain computed tomography (CT), while not necessary before normal general anesthesia, is essential before mECT to check for the presence of intracranial occupying lesions.

1.4.3 Check of Medications

Many patients requiring mECT have drug-resistant conditions and therefore receive pharmacotherapy with typical or atypical antipsychotics and/or many types of antidepressants. In patients with drug-resistant conditions, medications—not only current but also past—should be checked in detail, as follows.

Table 1.4 Pre-procedural examination list

1.	Minimum requirements
	Chest and abdominal X-ray, ECG, brain CT, SpO2, laboratory examination (Alb, BUN, Cr, Na, K, Cl, AST, ALT, LDH, ChE, CPK, Glu, CRP, WBC, Hct, Hb, Plt, Hb-Ag, HCV-Ad, STS)
2.	Adequate requirements
	Brain-MTI, brain-MRA, EEG, SPECT, respiratory function, cardiac function, echocardiography, holter-ECG

1.5 Preparation for Anesthetic Management of mECT

Although the duration of anesthetic management for mECT is short, preparation must be the same as for any normal general anesthesia, including instructions regarding nil by mouth and internal use as well as venous lines and various monitors.

1.5.1 Monitoring

Table 1.5 lists recommendations on monitoring during anesthesia published by the Japanese Society of Anesthesiologists [15]. This monitoring is necessary to quickly evaluate physiological changes as a result of mECT.

1.5.2 Instructions Regarding Nil by Mouth

As described, patients requiring mECT may have bowel dysfunction, meaning aspiration is a risk during anesthesia. Therefore, enough time should be provided for nil by mouth to take effect; ideally, patients are required to stop eating from 9 pm the day before receiving mECT and to stop drinking 6 h before mECT.

1.5.3 Instructions Regarding Internal Use

All medications, except cardiovascular agents, must be discontinued for a certain period before mECT. The timing for stopping each drug is shown in Table 1.6. In some patients, if discontinuing medication is difficult, internal use may be continued until 1 day before the procedure.

Table 1.5 Recommended monitoring during anesthesia, published by the Japanese Society of Anesthesiologists

①	An anesthesiologist must remain by the patient's side during anesthesia and must constantly observe the patient
②	Oxygenation must be checked via skin color and/or pulse oximeter
③	Evaluation of respiration via thoracic motion, capnography, or ventilation monitor is recommended
④	Hemodynamics must be checked via heart sound, palpation of the arteries, or pulse oximeter
	Electrocardiogram must be monitored
	Blood pressure must be checked at 5-min intervals
	Invasive arterial pressure measurement may be required as necessary
⑤	Body temperature must be checked
⑥	Degree of neuromuscular block may be checked as necessary

Table 1.6 Timing of discontinuation of each drug before mECT

	Timing of discontinuation	Notes
Atypical antipsychotics (phenothiazine, butyrophenone, etc.)	2 weeks before mECT	The α-receptor-blocking function of atypical antipsychotics may induce hypotension during anesthesia
Monoamine oxidase inhibitors	10 weeks before mECT	Hypertensive crisis may occur if an indirect vasoconstrictor such as ephedrine is administered in patients receiving monoamine oxidase inhibitors
Lithium carbonate	24 h before mECT	Lithium may be a risk factor for cognitive deficit after general anesthesia. Lithium may also increase muscle relaxation by suxamethonium or rocuronium
Anticonvulsants	2–3 times the half-life of each anticonvulsant before mECT	Seizure threshold may be increased in patients receiving anticonvulsant therapy. Phenytoin and carbamazepine may reduce muscle relaxation properties of non-depolarizing muscle relaxants

1.6 Pre-procedure Assessment of Patients with Depression [16–27]

In mECT for patients with depression, a detailed investigation of pharmacotherapy, cardiovascular disease, QT prolongation, and diabetes, among others, is necessary before the procedure.

1.6.1 Pharmacotherapy

A list of medications for depression is shown in Table 1.7. Antidepressants vary widely, with the first line usually being selective serotonin reuptake inhibitors (SSRIs), then tricyclic antidepressants (TCAs) or tetracyclic antidepressants (TeCAs) may be selected for moderate to severe depression. Patients requiring mECT are usually receiving pharmacotherapy with TCAs or TeCAs. Table 1.8 lists details to note regarding these medications.

1.6.2 Cardiovascular Disease

Patients with depression have a high risk of cardiovascular disease, regardless of pharmacotherapy; reasons for this are shown in Table 1.9. Depression itself is

Table 1.7 List of medications for depression

First generation (tricyclic)	Imipramine, amitriptyline, trimipramin, nortriptyline, clomipramine
Second generation (tricyclic)	Amoxapine, lofepramine, dosulepin
Second generation (tetracyclic)	Maprotiline, mianserin, setiptiline
Second generation (others)	Trazodone, sulpiride
Third generation (SSRI)	Fluvoxamine, paroxetine
Fourth generation (SNRI)	Milnacipran, duloxetine
Fourth generation (NaSSA)	Mirtazapine

Table 1.8 Points to note about tricyclic antidepressants and tetracyclic antidepressants

1.	Risk for myocardial infarction
2.	Tachycardia and increase in myocardial oxygen consumption due to cholinergic effects
3.	Hemodynamic events, such as hypotension, reduction of cardiac contractility, or sudden death, among others, because of depletion of noradrenaline at nerve endings and down-regulation of β-adrenergic receptor
4.	QT prolongation and risk for Torsade de Pointes

Table 1.9 Reasons for cardiovascular diseases in patients with depression

1.	Risk for arrhythmia due to heart rate variability by depression
2.	Risk for myocardial infarction due to platelet aggregation by dysregulation of the serotonin system
3.	Acceleration of atherosclerotic lesions due to enhancement of the immune system
4.	Deterioration of lifestyle, high smoking rates, alcohol polydipsia, and decrease in physical activities, among others, related to reduced motivation for healthy behaviors
5.	Hypotension, decrease in cardiac contractile force and prolongation of QT interval due to tricyclic antidepressant and tetracyclic antidepressant
6.	High risk for diabetes

considered a risk factor for ischemic heart disease and myocardial infarction. A report has indicated that the TCAs and TeCAs increase the risk for cardiovascular events. On the other hand, SSRIs are safe for use in ischemic heart disease and may provide a preventive effect for cardiovascular events.

1.6.3 QT Prolongation

It is well known that TCAs and TeCAs increase the QT interval, resulting in Torsade de Pointes. Therefore, the QT interval must be evaluated carefully before mECT. Table 1.10 shows special risks regarding QT prolongation in patients receiving TCAs or TeCAs. SSRIs and serotonin-norepinephrine reuptake inhibitors (SNRIs) may pose less risk than TCAs and TeCAs.

Table 1.10 Special risks regarding QT prolongation

1.	Congenital long QT syndrome
2.	Heart failure
3.	Bradycardia
4.	Electrolyte imbalance
5.	Excessive administration of psychotropic
6.	Excessive administration of antidepressant
7.	Female
8.	Elderly
9.	Liver or renal dysfunction

1.6.4 Diabetes

Patients receiving antidepressants may be at risk for diabetes. A report has indicated that taking antidepressants for more than 2 years increases the risk of diabetes. Furthermore, in patients with diabetes and depression, glycemic control may be unstable, resulting in high mortality. Therefore, risk of diabetes in a patient with depression must be evaluated before the procedure. Blood glucose level must be controlled carefully during mECT therapy.

1.7 Pre-procedure Assessment of Patients with Schizophrenia [28–42]

Patients diagnosed with schizophrenia and requiring mECT may also have many physical diseases. Furthermore, the presence of these diseases may go unnoticed because communication with patients with schizophrenia may be difficult.

Patients with schizophrenia are usually known to have a higher risk for perioperative complications than healthy subjects. Table 1.11 shows possible problems that may occur during mECT therapy.

1.7.1 Pharmacotherapy

Table 1.12 shows a medication list for schizophrenia. Antipsychotics are varied and are classified as typical or atypical antipsychotics. Usually, patients requiring mECT have been receiving multiple typical antipsychotics over a long period. Furthermore, these patients have often also received other types of medications, such as antiparkinson agents to prevent parkinsonism. These agents have side effects such as ileus, hydrodipsia, and cognitive decline, among others.

Table 1.11 Problems during mECT therapy in patients with schizophrenia

1.	Difficulty communicating
2.	Poor physical status
3.	Many physical problems
4.	High risk of restlessness after general anesthesia
5.	High risk of bowel dysfunction
6.	Synergistic effect between psychotropics and anesthetics
7.	Endocrine dysfunction
8.	Immune dysfunction
9.	Thermoregulatory dysfunction
10.	Diabetes
11.	QT prolongation

Table 1.12 List of medications for schizophrenia

Phenothiazine	Chlorpromazine, levomepromazine, propericiazine, perphenazine
Butyrophenone	Haloperidol, bromperidol, pipamperone, moperone, timiperone
Diphenylbutylpiperidine	Pimozide
Benzamide	Sulpiride, sultopride, nemonapride,
Thiepine	Zotepine
Indole	Oxypertine
Iminodibenzyl	Clocapramine
Iminodibenzyl	Clocapramine, mosapramine
Benzisoxazole	Risperidone
Thienobenzodiazepine	Olanzapine
Dibenzothiazepine	Quetiapine
Benzisothiazole	Perospirone
Quinolinone	Aripiprazole

1.7.2 Difficult Communication

Many patients with schizophrenia have problems with communication, resulting in difficult pre-procedure evaluations. Furthermore, their history of schizophrenia is usually long, so it may be difficult to obtain detailed information from their medical records.

1.7.3 QT Prolongation

It is well known that pharmacotherapy in patients with schizophrenia can increase the QT interval in electrocardiograms. QT prolongation is a risk for Torsade de Pointes; therefore, the QT interval must be evaluated carefully before the procedure. Some reports have indicated that events regarding Torsade de Pointes and sudden death are twice as high in patients receiving typical antipsychotics as in healthy subjects. The risk for QT prolongation may be lower with atypical antipsychotics than with typical antipsychotics.

1.7.4 Bowel Dysfunction

Bowel function is potentially decreased in patients with schizophrenia and should be checked in the pre-procedure evaluation. However, this may not be easy in patients who have difficulty communicating. These patients may require abdominal X-ray to evaluate bowel function and a longer period of nil by mouth.

1.7.5 Synergy Between Psychotropics and Anesthetics

The alpha adrenergic receptor-blocking action of psychotropics (especially chlorpromazine) may result in hypotension during anesthesia because of their synergy with anesthetics.

1.7.6 Endocrinopathy

As psychotropics potentially modulate the central cholinergic and serotonergic systems, blood levels of both noradrenaline and cortisol in patients with schizophrenia are potentially lower than in control subjects. Various stimuli increase these hormones in patients with schizophrenia. For these reasons, mECT carries the risk of hypotension.

1.7.7 Pulmonary Disease

It is well known that patients with schizophrenia may experience pneumonia and chronic bronchitis. There are two reasons for this: (1) the smoking rate in patients with schizophrenia is significant, at 75 %, and is three times higher than in healthy subjects; (2) psychotropics may result in a decreased cough reflex and gag reflex. Therefore, it is important to be aware of a risk of aspiration during and after mECT.

1.8 Management of Special Patient Populations for mECT [4, 43–48]

For special patient populations, it is crucial to assess the patient's condition, make an anesthesia plan, and prepare anesthesia carefully and according to individual needs.

1.8.1 Patients with Preexisting Cardiovascular Disease

To minimize a risk of myocardial ischemia, complications such as hypertension, angina pectoris, and diabetes, among others, must be well managed.

1. If blood pressure is unstable, pre-administration of nicardipine may be considered to prevent an hemodynamic response to mECT.
2. If the patient has coronary heart disease, pre-administration of a β-blocker is recommended to minimize an increase in oxygen consumption.
3. If the patient has bradycardia or sick sinus syndrome, pre-administration of atropine is recommended.
4. If the patient has an artificial cardiac pacemaker, the pacing mode must be changed to asynchronous before mECT and returned to the original mode after mECT.

1.8.2 Patients with Bowel Dysfunction

Long-term therapy with antipsychotics may lead to bowel dysfunction. Bowel function should be evaluated via abdominal X-ray, and if signs of bowel dysfunction, ileus, megacolon, etc. are observed, mECT rapid sequence induction with tracheal intubation should be performed or mECT should be postponed.

1.8.3 Patients with QT Prolongation

As previously mentioned, typical antipsychotics and antidepressants such as TCAs and TeCAs may increase the QT interval, resulting in Torsade de Pointes.

1.8.4 Patients with Neuroleptic Malignant Syndrome

Neuroleptic Malignant Syndrome (NMS) is a serious side effect produced by antipsychotics. Patients with NMS will manifest increases in temperature and serum creatine kinase levels after administration of a triggering drug. Nondepolarizing muscle relaxants, such as rocuronium, are recommended in place of succinylcholine in patients with NMS. If the patient is experiencing rhabdomyolysis, the mECT should be postponed except in emergency cases.

1.8.5 Patients with Cerebral Aneurysms

mECT induces abrupt changes in both systemic and cerebral hemodynamics. The cerebrovascular changes increase the wall stress in aneurysms, leading to enlargement or rupture. In patients suspected of having cerebral aneurysms, the selection of hypnotic anesthetics and the administration of a vasodilator before mECT is crucial to prevent hemodynamic changes.

The increase in cerebral blood flow velocity during mECT is generally less with propofol than with thiopental. Although nicardipine (0.02 m/kg) fails to block the increase in cerebral blood flow velocity associated with mECT, both nitroglycerine and β-blockers partially inhibit it.

1.8.6 Patients with Intracranial Mass Lesion

mECT provokes an increase in intracranial pressure, leading to serious conditions in patients with intracranial mass lesions. Special efforts should be made to reduce intracranial pressure by pretreating patients with steroids and diuretics. Hyperventilation before mECT may be effective in preventing it.

1.8.7 Pregnant Patients

Although mECT can successfully manage pregnancy-induced depression, there are some potential complications for both the mother (e.g., aspiration and premature labor) and the fetus (e.g., spontaneous abortion and death). If mECT is indicated in a pregnant patient, a trained obstetrician must remain by the patient's side, and the fetal heart rate must be monitored.

1.9 QT Dispersion and mECT [49, 50]

QT dispersion (QTD), defined as maximal QT interval minus minimal QT interval, on a 12-lead surface electrocardiogram reflects the regional heterogeneity of ventricular repolarization. Prolongation of the QTD is associated with an increased risk of ventricular arrhythmia and cardiovascular mortality. It is well known that the QTD is regulated not only by heart rate but also by autonomic tone.

QTD in patients with major depression has been reported as significantly larger than in healthy subjects (Fig. 1.1), and electrical stimulus during mECT has been reported to induce a further increase in the QTD (Fig. 1.2). This phenomenon was

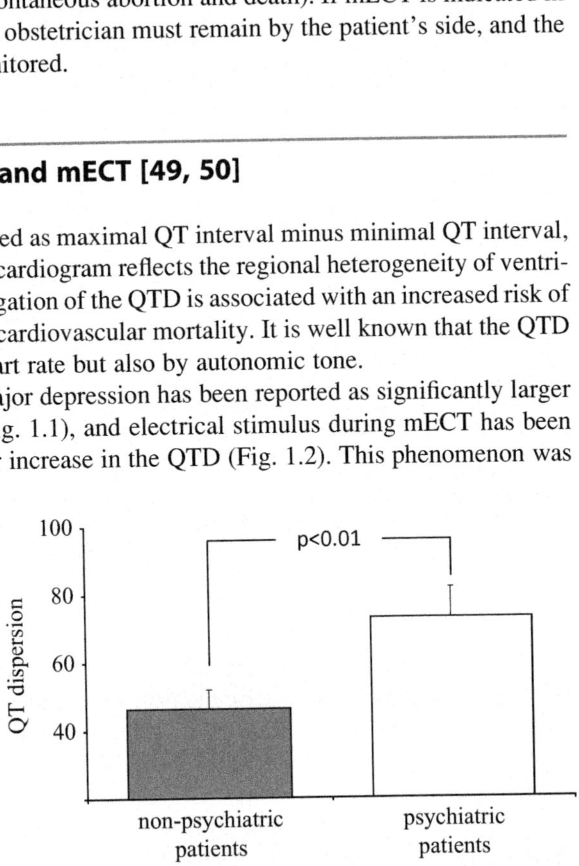

Fig. 1.1 QTc dispersion in psychiatric and non-psychiatric patients QTc dispersion in psychiatric patients was significantly larger than in non-psychiatric patients ($p < 0.05$)

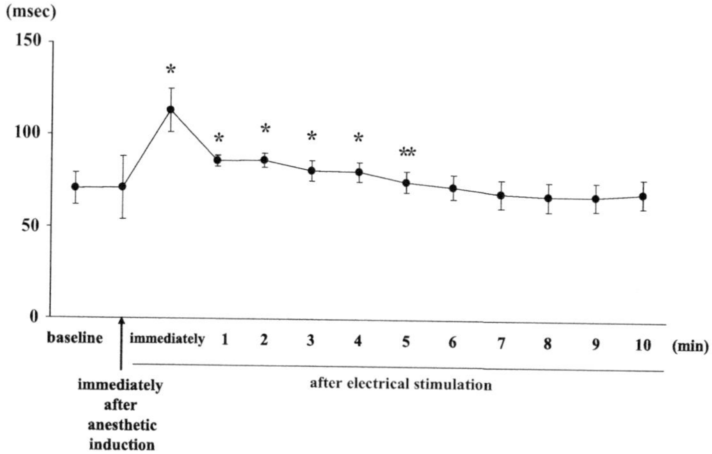

Fig. 1.2 Change in QTc dispersion during mECT therapy
QTc dispersion significantly increased immediately after electrical stimulus

more obvious in elderly patients with major depression. Therefore, patients with major depression should be considered at high risk for arrhythmia during mECT.

1.10 Summary

Management of anesthesia for mECT may be more difficult than expected because of the patient's condition (which may include physical complications), the influence of medications that patients requiring mECT may be taking, and the rapid effect of electrical stimulus. Therefore, the assessment and preparation of each patient is crucial before mECT to prevent serious problems.

References

1. Khan A, Mirolo MH, Hughes D, Bierut L. Electroconvulsive therapy. Psychiatr Clin North Am. 1993;16:497–513.
2. Thompson JW, Weiner RD, Myers CP. Use of ECT in the United States in 1975, 1980, and 1986. Am J Psychiatry. 1994;151:1657–61.
3. American Psychiatric Association Committee on Electroconvulsive Therapy. The practice of electroconvulsive therapy. 2nd ed. Washington, DC: American Psychiatric Association; 2001.
4. Ding Z, White PF. Anesthesia for electroconvulsive therapy. Anesth Analg. 2002;94:1351–64.
5. Pagnin D, de Queiroz V, Pini S, Cassano GB. Efficacy of ECT in depression: a meta-analytic review. J ECT. 2004;20:13–20.
6. Kellner CH, Tobias KG, Jakubowski LM, Ali Z, Istafanous RM. Electroconvulsive therapy for an urgent social indication. J ECT. 2009;25:274–5.
7. The American Psychiatric Association Task Force on Electroconvulsive Therapy. Ther practice of electroconvulsive therapy: recommendations for treatment, training, and privileging: a

task force report of the American Psychiatric Association. Washington, DC: American Psychiatric Association; 1990. p. 6.
8. O'Flaherty D, Husain MM, Moore M, Wolff TR, Sills S, Giesecke AH. Circulatory responses during electroconvulsive therapy. The comparative effects of placebo, esmolol and nitroglycerin. Anaesthesia. 1992;47:563–7.
9. Weinger MB, Partridge BL, Hauger R, Mirow A. Prevention of the cardiovascular and neuroendocrine response to electroconvulsive therapy: I. Effectiveness of pretreatment regimens on hemodynamics. Anesth Analg. 1991;73:556–62.
10. Weinger MB, Partridge BL, Hauger R, Mirow A, Brown M. Prevention of the cardiovascular and neuroendocrine response to electroconvulsive therapy: II. Effects of pretreatment regimens on catecholamines, ACTH, vasopressin, and cortisol. Anesth Analg. 1991;73:563–9.
11. Partridge BL, Weinger MB, Hauger R. Is the cardiovascular response to electroconvulsive therapy due to the electricity or the subsequent convulsion? Anesth Analg. 1991;72:706–9.
12. Saito S. Anesthesia management for electroconvulsive therapy: hemodynamic and respiratory management. J Anesth. 2005;19:142–9.
13. Simpson KH, Lynch L. Anaesthesia and electroconvulsive therapy (ECT). Anaesthesia. 1998; 53:615–7.
14. Lyndon W, Wilson C. Anesthesia for electroconvulsive therapy – time for a review? Brain Stimul. 2015;8:985–6.
15. http://www.anesth.or.jp/guide/pdf/monitor2.pdf
16. Joynt KE, Whellan DJ, O'Connor CM. Depression and cardiovascular disease: mechanisms of interaction. Biol Psychiatry. 2003;54:248–61.
17. Wulsin LR, Vaillant GE, Wells VE. A systematic review of the mortality of depression. Psychosom Med. 1999;61:6–17.
18. Lichtman JH, Bigger JT Jr, Blumenthal JA, Frasure-Smith N, Kaufmann PG, Lespérance F, Mark DB, Sheps DS, Taylor CB, Froelicher ES. AHA science advisory. Depression and coronary heart disease. Recommendations for screening, referral, and treatment. A science advisory from the American Heart Association Prevention Committee to the Council on Cardiovascular Nursing, Council on Clinical Cardiology, Council on Epidemiology and Prevention, and Interdisciplinary Council on Quality of Care Outcomes Research. Endorsed by the American Psychiatric Association. Prog Cardiovasc Nurs. 2009;24:19–26.
19. Lichtman JH, Bigger JT Jr, Blumenthal JA, Frasure-Smith N, Kaufmann PG, Lespérance F, Mark DB, Sheps DS, Taylor CB, Froelicher ES, American Heart Association Prevention Committee of the Council on Cardiovascular Nursing; American Heart Association Council on Clinical Cardiology, American Heart Association Council on Epidemiology and Prevention, American Heart Association Interdisciplinary Council on Quality of Care and Outcomes Research, American Psychiatric Association. Depression and coronary heart disease: recommendations for screening, referral, and treatment: a science advisory from the American Heart Association Prevention Committee of the Council on Cardiovascular Nursing, Council on Clinical Cardiology, Council on Epidemiology and Prevention, and Interdisciplinary Council on Quality of Care and Outcomes Research: endorsed by the American Psychiatric Association. Circulation. 2008;118:1768–75.
20. Braverman B, McCarthy RJ, Ivankovich AD. Vasopressor challenges during chronic MAOI or TCA treatment in anesthetized dogs. Life Sci. 1987;40:2587–95.
21. Drugs for psychiatric disorders. Med Lett Drugs Ther. 1991;33:43–50.
22. Ray WA, Meredith S, Thapa PB, Hall K, Murray KT. Cyclic antidepressants and the risk of sudden cardiac death. Clin Pharmacol Ther. 2004;75:234–41.
23. Cohen HW, Gibson G, Alderman MH. Excess risk of myocardial infarction in patients treated with antidepressant medications: association with use of tricyclic agents. Am J Med. 2000;108: 2–8.
24. Tata LJ, West J, Smith C, Farrington P, Card T, Smeeth L, Hubbard R. General population based study of the impact of tricyclic and selective serotonin reuptake inhibitor antidepressants on the risk of acute myocardial infarction. Heart. 2005;91:465–71.
25. Sicouri S, Antzelevitch C. Sudden cardiac death secondary to antidepressant and antipsychotic drugs. Expert Opin Drug Saf. 2008;7:181–94.

26. Andersohn F, Schade R, Suissa S, Garbe E. Long-term use of antidepressants for depressive disorders and the risk of diabetes mellitus. Am J Psychiatry. 2009;166:591–8.
27. Katon W, Fan MY, Unützer J, Taylor J, Pincus H, Schoenbaum M. Depression and diabetes: a potentially lethal combination. J Gen Intern Med. 2008;23:1571–5.
28. Ray WA, Meredith S, Thapa PB, Meador KG, Hall K, Murray KT. Antipsychotics and the risk of sudden cardiac death. Arch Gen Psychiatry. 2001;58:1161–7.
29. Goldman LS. Medical illness in patients with schizophrenia. J Clin Psychiatry. 1999;60:s10–5.
30. Dworkin RH. Pain insensitivity in schizophrenia: a neglected phenomenon and some implications. Schizophr Bull. 1994;20:235–48.
31. Adler LE, Griffith JM. Concurrent medical illness in the schizophrenic patient. Epidemiology, diagnosis, and management. Schizophr Res. 1991;4:91–107.
32. Haddad PM, Anderson IM. Antipsychotic-related QTc prolongation, torsade de pointes and sudden death. Drugs. 2002;62:1649–71.
33. Glassman AH. Schizophrenia, antipsychotic drugs, and cardiovascular disease. J Clin Psychiatry. 2005;66:s5–10.
34. Glassman AH, Bigger Jr JT. Antipsychotic drugs: prolonged QTc interval, torsade de pointes, and sudden death. Am J Psychiatry. 2001;158:1774–82.
35. Kuehn BM. FDA warns antipsychotic drugs may be risky for elderly. JAMA. 2005;293:2462.
36. de Leon J, Diaz FJ, Rogers T, Browne D, Dinsmore L. Initiation of daily smoking and nicotine dependence in schizophrenia and mood disorders. Schizophr Res. 2002;56:47–54.
37. Copeland LA, Mortensen EM, Zeber JE, Pugh MJ, Restrepo MI, Dalack GW. Pulmonary disease among inpatient decedents: impact of schizophrenia. Prog Neuropsychopharmacol Biol Psychiatry. 2007;31:720–6.
38. Chafetz L, White MC, Collins-Bride G, Nickens J. The poor general health of the severely mentally ill: impact of schizophrenic diagnosis. Community Ment Health J. 2005;41:169–84.
39. Nagamine T. Serum substance P levels in patients with chronic schizophrenia treated with typical or atypical antipsychotics. Neuropsychiatr Dis Treat. 2008;4:289–94.
40. Kudoh A, Katagai H, Takase H, Takazawa T. Effect of preoperative discontinuation of antipsychotics in schizophrenic patients on outcome during and after anaesthesia. Eur J Anaesthesiol. 2004;21:414–6.
41. Kudoh A, Ishihara H, Matsuki A. Pituitary-adrenal and parasympathetic function in chronic schizophrenic patients with postoperative ileus or hypotension. Neuropsychobiology. 1999;39:125–30.
42. Kudoh A, Kudo T, Ishihara H, Matsuki A. Depressed pituitary-adrenal response to surgical stress in chronic schizophrenic patients. Neuropsychobiology. 1997;36:112–6.
43. Applegate RJ. Diagnosis and management of ischemic heart disease in the patient scheduled to undergo electroconvulsive therapy. Convuls Ther. 1997;13:128–244.
44. Saito S, Kadoi Y, Iriuchijima N, Obata H, Arai K, Morita T, Goto F. Reduction of cerebral hyperemia with anti-hypertensive medication after electroconvulsive therapy. Can J Anaesth. 2000;47:767–74.
45. Wijeratne C, Shome S. Electroconvulsive therapy and subdural hemorrhage. J ECT. 1999;15:275–9.
46. Nisijima K, Ishiguro T. Electroconvulsive therapy for the treatment of neuroleptic malignant syndrome with psychotic symptoms: a report of five cases. J ECT. 1999;15:158–63.
47. Kelly D, Brull SJ. Neuroleptic malignant syndrome and mivacurium: a safe alternative to succinylcholine? Can J Anaesth. 1994;41:845–9.
48. Echevarría Moreno M, Martin Muñoz J, Sanchez Valderrabanos J, Vázquez Gutierrez T. Electroconvulsive therapy in the first trimester of pregnancy. J ECT. 1998;14:251–4.
49. Tezuka N, Egawa H, Fukagawa D, Yamaguchi S, Hamaguchi S, Kitajima T, Minami J. Assessment of QT interval and QT dispersion during electroconvulsive therapy using computerized measurements. J ECT. 2010;26:41–6.
50. Yamaguchi S, Nagao M, Ikeda T, Fukagawa D, Kimura Y, Kitajima T, Minami J. QT dispersion and rate-corrected QT dispersion during electroconvulsive therapy in elderly patients. J ECT. 2011;27:183–8.

Comprehensive Monitoring During Procedures Under Reasonable Anesthetic Control

2

Yoshihiko Demoto

Abstract

It is quite important to induce qualitatively effective seizure electroencephalogram (EEG) under proper sedation, respiratory management, and cardiovascular stability for safe and therapeutically effective electroconvulsive therapy (ECT).

However, avoidable circulatory and respiratory complications during ECT still occur. Besides, failure to induce qualitatively effective seizures is still relatively common.

Therefore, it is necessary to develop methodologically rational anesthesia management based on proper and comprehensive judgment of multifarious information from various monitors and computer simulation software, such as transitional changes in plasma and effect-site concentrations of intravenous anesthetics, to increase the safety and efficacy of ECT.

In this chapter, we will introduce our practical anesthesia procedures for ECT and compare them to those traditionally used. Moreover, we will expound the significance to the optimal use of various monitors, devices, and computer simulation software, which are already brought into clinical application, while explaining their special characteristics and important points to notice.

Furthermore, we will summarize current methods for qualitative evaluation of seizure EEG.

Keywords

Electroconvulsive therapy • Effect-site concentration • End-tidal carbon dioxide tension • Bispectral index monitoring • Evaluation of seizure

---

Y. Demoto (✉)
Department of Anesthesia, Hiroshima Haruka Clinic, 2-12-8-404, Shinonome, 734-0022 Minami-ku, Hiroshima, Japan
e-mail: yoshihikodemoto@yahoo.co.jp

S. Saito (ed.), *Anesthesia Management for Electroconvulsive Therapy*,
DOI 10.1007/978-4-431-55717-3_2

2.1 Background and Our Practical Approach

Electroconvulsive therapy (ECT) remains a requisite treatment for serious and drug-refractory psychiatric disorders. However, there are still many methodological issues to consider for successful ECT.

2.1.1 Current Problems in ECT

Patient safety depends on the induction of qualitatively effective seizures under proper sedation, respiratory management, and cardiovascular stability [1]. However, it is often difficult to meet all conditions, mainly because of differences in individual patients or resulting from anesthesia management (Fig. 2.1).

2.1.1.1 Factors Interfering with Qualitatively Effective Seizure Induction Because of Differences in Individual Patients

Patients scheduled for ECT may continue taking antidepressants or major tranquilizers. Further, while it is generally recommended that antiepileptic drugs used as mood stabilizer or benzodiazepine-descent medicines having anxiety-relieving or sleep-assisting agents should be terminated, these may be suspended

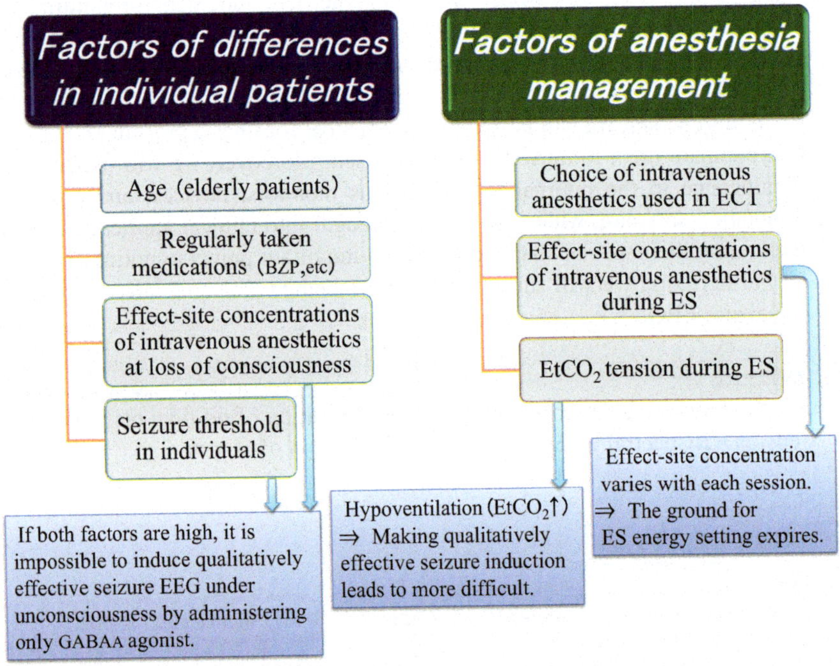

Fig. 2.1 Factors interfering with qualitatively effective seizure induction

only shortly before first ECT session. Thus, the residual anticonvulsant effects of these medications may hinder qualitatively effective seizure induction.

Besides, many intravenous anesthetic agents used for ECT, particularly $GABA_A$ agonists, such as propofol and thiopental, have anticonvulsive properties, and their sedative doses differ among individual patients. In general, the higher are the effect-site concentrations at a loss of consciousness, the greater are the anticonvulsant effects.

Furthermore, it is known that individual seizure threshold increases with age, making qualitatively effective seizure induction even more difficult in some elderly patients, and there are also great individual differences in seizure threshold regardless of age [2].

Thus, in individuals whose effect-site concentrations of intravenous anesthetics at loss of consciousness and seizure threshold are both high, it may be impossible to induce qualitatively effective seizures under unconsciousness using $GABA_A$ agonists alone.

2.1.1.2 Factors Interfering with Qualitatively Effective Seizure Induction Resulting from Anesthesia Management

Traditional procedures of anesthesia for ECT often adopt either propofol or thiopental. Although propofol pharmacokinetics well fit the three-compartment model and is suitable for target-controlled infusion (TCI) [3], it has a stronger anticonvulsant effect than thiopental at the equivalent level of sedation. In contrast, the reality is that thiopental effect-site concentration cannot be predicted by computer simulation over a longer period for TCI because of its slow clearance.

Moreover, although single-dose administration of intravenous anesthetics is common in the traditional anesthesia for ECT, transitional changes in effect-site concentrations are sharp with any intravenous anesthetics (Fig. 2.2). Therefore, unless it is possible to strictly manage the course of time from single-dose administration to electrical stimulation (ES), effect-site concentrations and concomitant anticonvulsant effects at the time of ES will vary with each session, creating greater uncertainty for setting ES energy.

Further, it is known that qualitatively effective seizure induction is more difficult if the patient is under hypoventilation at the time of ES.

2.1.1.3 Great Responsibility of Anesthesiologists During ECT

To induce qualitatively effective seizures, anesthesiologists need to completely understand the factors, all of which can increase the difficulty of safely and reliably inducing therapeutic effective seizures. Thus, anesthesiologists are compelled to develop improved procedures with methodological rationality and enhanced safety.

Though not an easy task, the optimal use of current physiological monitoring devices and computer simulation technology for monitoring transitional changes in plasma and effect-site concentrations of intravenous anesthetics can greatly aid in achieving these goals.

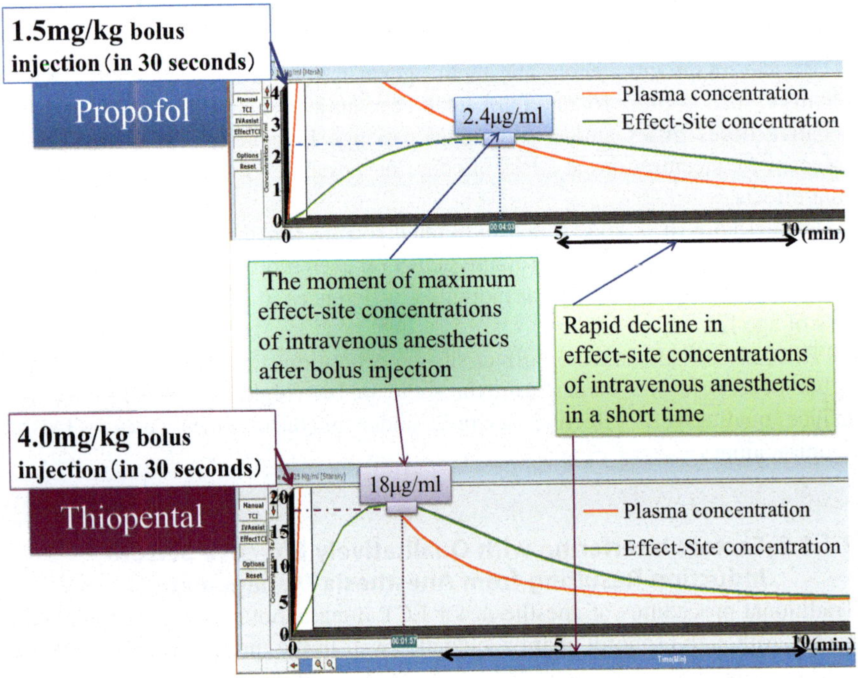

Fig. 2.2 Acute changes in effect-site concentrations of propofol and thiopental

2.1.2 Our Comprehensive Approach to Rational Anesthesia Management and Monitoring During ECT

As discussed, there are some real limitations to the traditional procedure of anesthesia for ECT. More rationale techniques and methodologies for administration of intravenous anesthetics will allow comprehensive monitoring and management of breathing, sedation, and circulation during ECT to improve the quality of anesthesia for safe and successful ECT.

2.1.2.1 Methodology for Intravenous Anesthetic Administration During ECT, Focused on Effect-Site Concentrations of Propofol and Remifentanil

Our basic strategy relies on the mutually re-enforcing properties of propofol and remifentanil to enhance sedation while reducing the anticonvulsant potential of anesthesia.

First, we referred to studies conducted on the mutually potentiating effects of propofol and remifentanil and the correlation with sedation level [4–6], as well as our own clinical experience.

We then prepared eight anesthetic settings (groups A – F, A′, and S) for effect-site concentrations of propofol and remifentanil during ES using TIVA trainer ver.8

		Propofol (μg/ml)	Remifentanil (ng/ml)
	Group S	2.0	30
	Group A'	1.5	30
Basic setting →	**Group A**	**1.5**	**20**
	Group B	1.0	20
	Group C	0.7	20
	Group D	0.5	20
	Group E	0.2	30
	Group F	0	30

Fig. 2.3 Effect-site concentration settings of propofol and remifentanil
TCI and SAI for "the same individuals," under "the same conditions" (with no previous injection of special psychotropic and no physical change including cardiac function), and using "the same simulation software."
Considering age, physical condition (cardiac function, etc.), BMI, regularly taken medications, and choosing from among group A, B, and C at the first session,
if sedation level is not sufficient according to patient's response and BIS-EEG features, effect-site concentration settings of propofol and remifentanil are altered to group A' or group S

(European Society of Intravenous Anesthesia). On this occasion, anesthesia is induced by TCI of propofol with effect-site concentrations of 0–2.0 μg/ml and simulation-assisted infusion (SAI) of remifentanil with effect-site concentrations of 20 or 30 ng/ml (Figs. 2.3 and 2.4).

2.1.2.2 Our Practical Procedure for Anesthesia and Electrical Stimulation (ES)

We developed a procedure during ECT including anesthesia and ES thanks to various monitoring devices and based on our eight effect-site concentration settings of propofol and remifentanil with approval by the local ethics committee of Kouseikai Kusatsu Hospital in Hiroshima, Japan.

- After sufficient preoxygenation and precurarization (2–3 mg rocuronium), propofol anesthesia is induced by TCI, remifentanil by SAI, choosing from among our eight effect-site concentration settings of propofol and remifentanil (Fig. 2.3).
- After loss of response to name calling and eyelash reflex, and after confirming EEG features of Bi-Spectral Index (BIS-EEG features) to ensure that consciousness is not clear using BIS monitor (BIS A-2000 XP; Aspect Medical), 0.8 mg/kg rocuronium is administered intravenously.
- Laryngeal mask airway (LMA) or endotracheal intubation is performed after confirming sufficient muscular relaxation using acceleromyography: train-of-four fade (TOF-Watch, TOF-2100; NIHON KOHDEN). End-tidal CO_2 ($EtCO_2$)

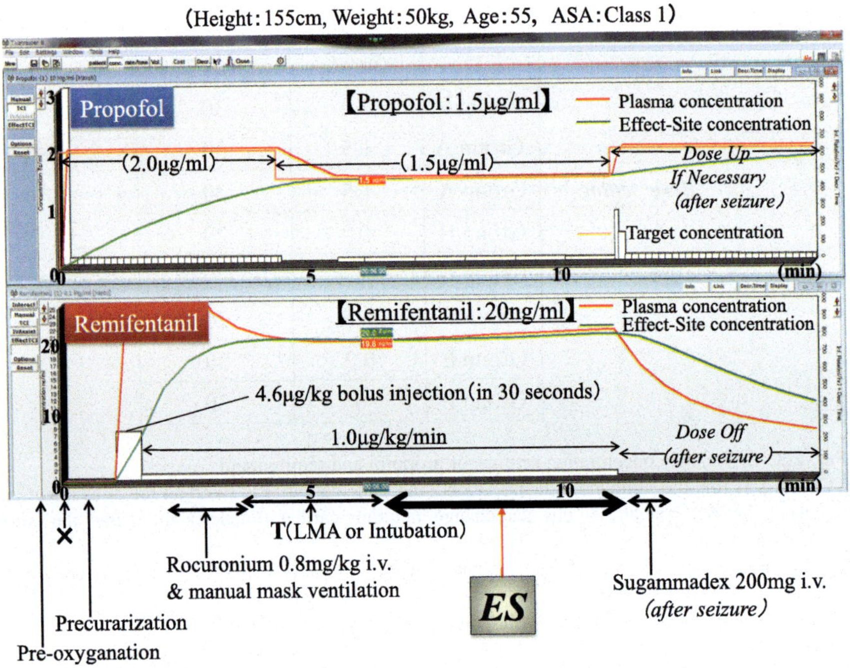

Fig. 2.4 Time course of anesthesia and electrical stimulation (Group A)

tension is maintained at 30–34 mmHg with the pressure control ventilation volume-guaranteed (PCV-VG) mode until ES.

- Continuous electrocardiography (ECG), noninvasive arterial blood pressure (NIBP) monitoring, pulse oximetry, capnography, TOF ratio monitoring, and BIS-EEG monitoring are conducted throughout the procedure.
- After sufficient muscular relaxation is confirmed using TOF-Watch, adequate sedation level according to BIS-EEG features is confirmed, and the expected hemodynamic changes associated with the target concentrations of propofol and remifentanil are observed, we confirm whether we are able to keep the effect-site concentrations of propofol and remifentanil at nearly fixed concentrations by TCI and SAI using TIVA trainer ver.8, and only then is ES applied to the bilateral temporal using Thymatron System IV (Somatics Inc., USA) (Figs. 2.5 and 2.6).
- Seizure EEG is continuously recorded from sensors attached to the bilateral forehead using the Thymatron System IV, and the qualitative evaluation of seizure EEG is performed.
- When seizure EEG is qualitatively judged as invalid, ES energy is modified concurrently with the effect-site concentration settings of propofol and remifentanil. Usually, ES of 1.5-fold greater energy is applied after blood pressure and heart rate have returned approximately to baseline (before the

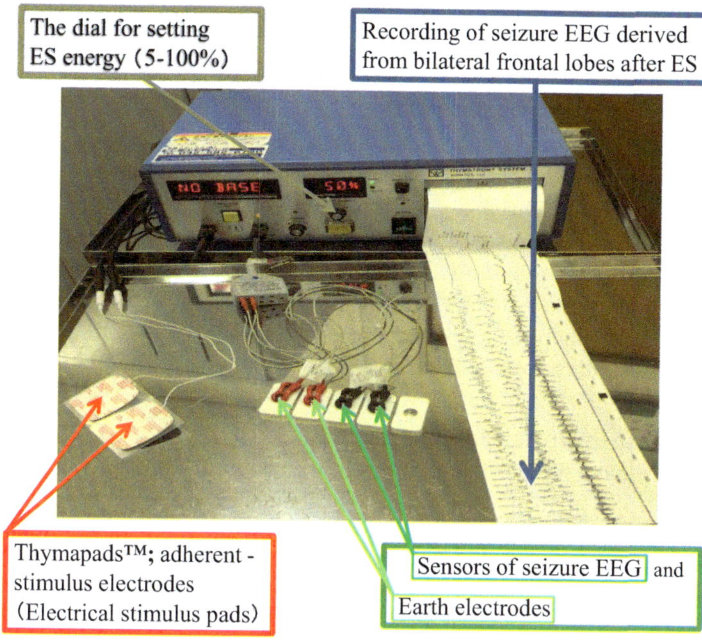

Fig. 2.5 Details of the Thymatron System IV

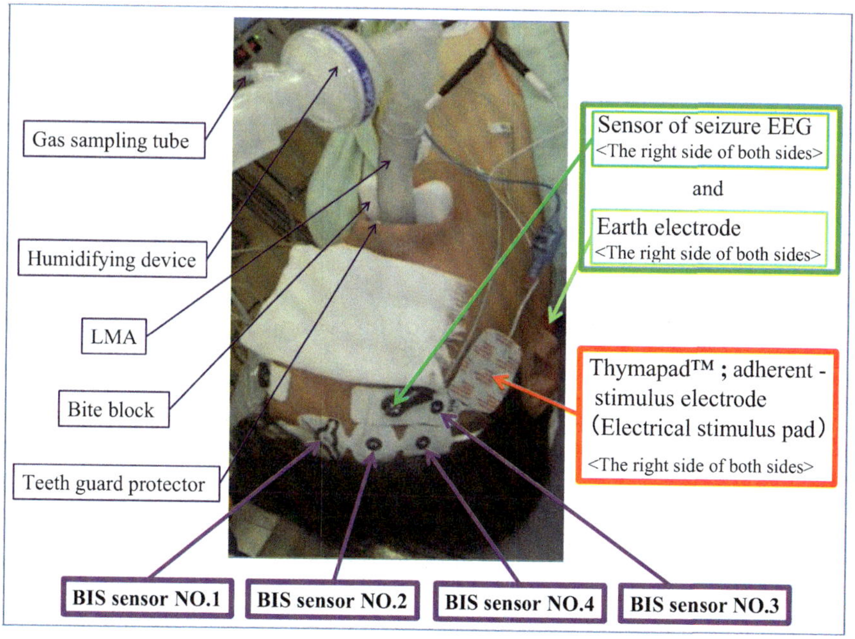

Fig. 2.6 Positions of sensors and electrodes of the BIS monitor and Thymatron System IV

first ES of the same session) and after confirming sedation level by BIS-EEG features and sufficient muscular relaxation by TOF-Watch.

- After induction of seizure EEG is qualitatively evaluated as valid, and confirming seizure end point and postictal suppression, we stop administration of remifentanil and suck in secretions gathering in the oral cavity and pharynx in parallel with the ventilator management by the PCV-VG mode (using LMA or endotracheal intubation) under sufficient muscular relaxation.
- Then, 200 mg Sugammadex is administered intravenously. After confirming sufficient recovery from muscular relaxation using TOF-Watch, we stop administration of propofol. After reappearance of spontaneous breathing, extubation is performed and increased levels of consciousness and breathing as well as circulatory stability are confirmed.

2.1.2.3 Postanesthesia Management for ECT

After patients leave the ECT unit, as a rule we continue administering oxygen for 2–3 h and perform frequent checks of physical remarks and vital signs as necessary. Longer monitoring may be indicated for patients in poor general condition, particularly those with comorbid heart or respiratory diseases.

2.2 Methodology of Intravenous Anesthetic Administration During ECT: Strict Control of Effect-Site Concentrations Using Computer Simulation Software

To achieve comprehensive monitoring and management of anesthesia for successful ECT, strict control of intravenous anesthetic concentrations is absolutely essential. Currently, computer simulation software for predicting transitional changes in plasma and effect-site concentrations is used extensively. We highlight important characteristics of our practical procedure, differences compared to traditional anesthesia during ECT, and risk management strategies.

2.2.1 Effect-Site Concentrations of Intravenous Anesthetics, Focused on the Timing of ES

Accurate estimates of the effect-site concentrations of intravenous anesthetics at the time of ES are critical for therapeutic effective seizure induction as $GABA_A$ agonists like propofol have anticonvulsive properties (Fig. 2.7).

2.2.1.1 Agenda for "Possible Reproducibility"

Firstly, as it is assumed that more than one session of ECT will be performed to one and the same individual, so reproducibility of effect-site concentrations, particularly of the (potent anticonvulsant) $GABA_A$ agonist, is critical for reliable seizure induction.

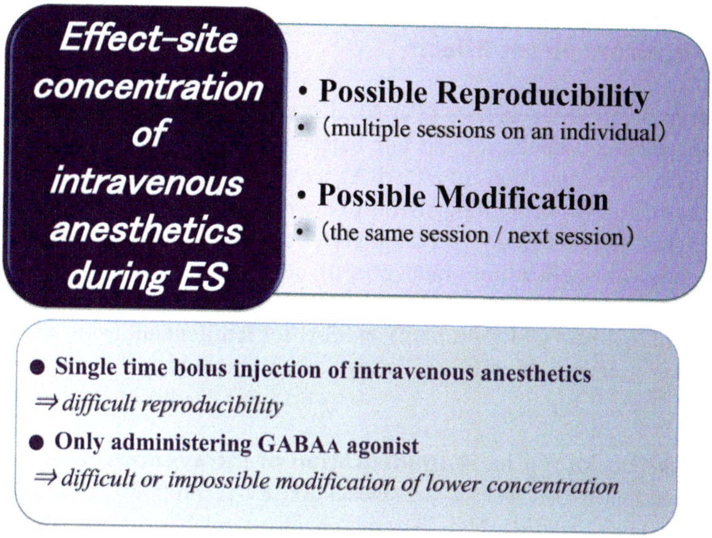

Fig. 2.7 Important matters concerning effect-site concentrations of intravenous anesthetics for successful ECT

In the traditional procedure of anesthesia during ECT, single-dose administration of intravenous anesthetics is common, in which case it is essential to strictly control the course of time between anesthesia induction and ES. To this end, it is indispensable that proper respiratory management, adequate sedation level, and cardiovascular stability are maintained, that all sensors are functioning properly, and that sufficient muscular relaxation has been achieved. However, variations and uncertainties in all of these factors can influence the timing of ES application.

For this reason, administration of intravenous anesthetics with control of effect-site concentrations (particularly with $GABA_A$ agonists) by TCI is considered more reliable.

2.2.1.2 Agenda for "Possible Modification"

In general, the greater the number of ECT sessions on the same individual, the higher the threshold for convulsions. Even with high energy ES, it may become difficult to induce qualitatively effective seizures.

Thus, it is critical that effect-site concentrations of intravenous anesthetics are modifiable. However, in case of anesthesia by $GABA_A$ agonist alone, lowering effect-site concentration is difficult or impossible because it increases the risk of the patient waking.

Therefore, addition of remifentanil is advantageous as it has no anticonvulsive properties in itself. Remifentanil is quickly metabolized by nonspecific esterase in human blood and tissues and exhibits rapid onset and recovery independent of liver and kidney function.

2.2.2 Balanced Use of Propofol and Remifentanil for Minimal Anticonvulsant Effects

For total intravenous anesthesia (TIVA), it is recommended that anesthesia management (sedation, analgesia, and circulatory control) should be achieved using well-balanced concentrations of a $GABA_A$ agonist and remifentanil to take advantage of the mutually potentiating effects of these intravenous anesthetics. However, if propofol is administered at the high effect-site concentrations used for routine general surgical applications, induction of qualitatively effective seizures may become impossible. To circumvent these problems, we apply a particular kind of TIVA for ECT with TCI for propofol and SAI for remifentanil using TIVA-trainer ver.8 shifted greatly to higher remifentanil and minimal propofol anesthesia.

2.2.2.1 Methodology for Administration of Intravenous Anesthetics

In our practical procedure of anesthesia for ECT, propofol TCI is aided by Diprifusor (TE-371; TERUMO), a commercially available syringe pump for TCI, and built-in Marsh's parameter included in TIVA trainer ver.8. Meanwhile, as the clinical use of commercially available syringe pumps for remifentanil TCI is not yet permitted in our country, remifentanil is administered intravenously via SAI with the help of a commonly used syringe pump (TE-332S; TERUMO) capable of continuous intravenous infusion at controlled velocity (μg/kg/min) and using Minto's parameter included in TIVA trainer ver.8.

For individuals with Body Mass Index (BMI) <22, the actual measured weight is applied for calculation of propofol TCI and remifentanil SAI. On the other hand, for individuals with BMI >22, actual body weight is applied for propofol, while lean body weight is applied for remifentanil before anesthesia is induced.

2.2.2.2 Criteria for Selecting from Among Our Anesthetic Settings: Choice of Effect-Site Concentration Settings of Propofol and Remifentanil

We first choose the anesthetic settings from among our three groups (A, B, or C) at the first ECT session, taking into consideration age, physical condition (cardiac function, etc.), BMI, and regularly taken medications (benzodiazepines, etc.).

The anesthetic settings are altered to group A' (Fig. 2.8) or group S respectively, if sedation level is insufficient according to patient's physical response and BIS-EEG features under the anesthetic setting of group A.

If we cannot induce qualitatively effective seizures under the anesthetic setting of group C during the first ECT session, ES of 1.5-fold greater energy is applied under the anesthetic setting of group D (after blood pressure and heart rate have returned approximately to baseline before the first ES of the same session, and after confirming sedation level by BIS-EEG features and sufficient muscular relaxation by TOF-Watch) (Fig. 2.9).

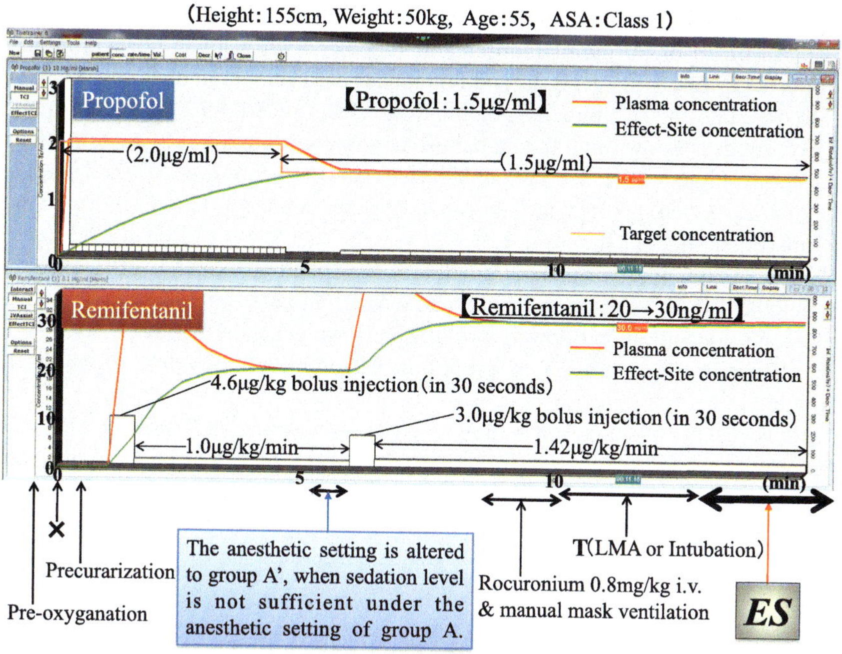

Fig. 2.8 Time course of anesthesia and electrical stimulation (Group A → A')

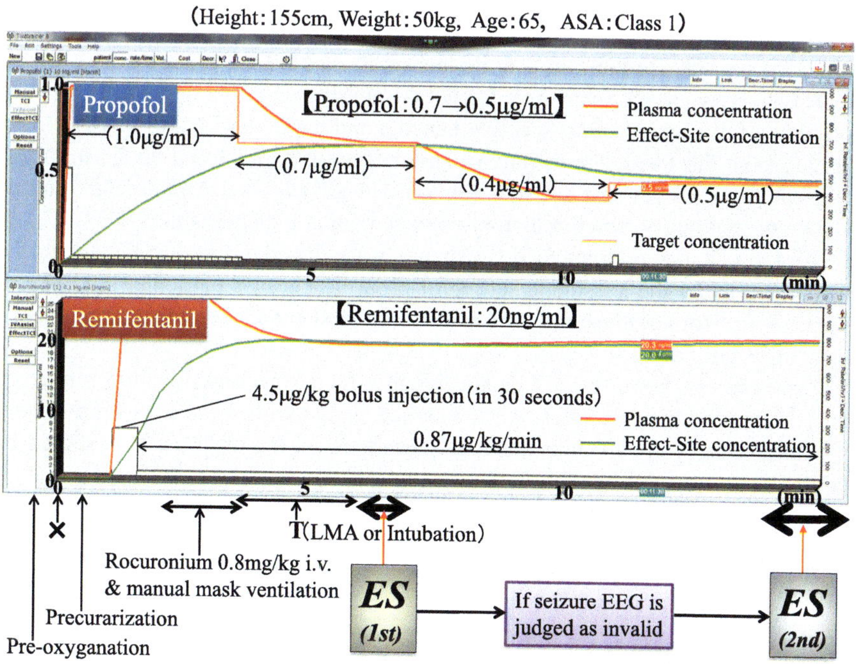

Fig. 2.9 Time course of anesthesia and electrical stimulation (Group C → D)

2.2.2.3 Important Considerations

The use of 20 or 30 ng/ml remifentanil together with a given concentration of propofol (groups S, A', A, B, C, and D) reduces cardiac output, blood pressure, and heart rate due to the mutually potentiating effects of propofol and remifentanil. Therefore, it is known that the actual effect-site concentration of propofol will be somewhat higher than the predicted effect-site concentration by the computer simulation, when taking into consideration the concept based on the three-compartment model [7].

And taking into consideration there are pharmacokinetic differences in individuals, it is an expected phenomenon as a matter of fact that the actual effect-site concentration of propofol is different with each individual, be it a setting for effect-site concentration of propofol: 1.0 μg/ml of the same group B, for example [8].

However, our practical procedure of anesthesia during ECT presupposes more than one session during a short term under conditions of TCI and SAI for the same individuals in the same conditions (with no previous injection of special psychotropic drugs and no physical change including cardiac function), using the same simulation software.

2.2.2.4 Special Considerations for the Anesthetic Setting of Group F Without Propofol

Although comprehensive safety is not yet established, we have encountered only a limited number of cases in which there was no other alternative but to perform ES at maximum energy under the anesthetic setting of group F to induce qualitatively effective seizures for their life-saving measures.

However, when ES is performed under the anesthetic setting of group F, we must provide a full account of prospective benefits and particular kind of possible risks arising from the specific procedure of anesthesia during ECT and obtain informed consent from all patients or their relatives in advance since particular kind of sedation, respiratory, and circulatory management is indispensable.

And yet, it has nothing to do with our recommendation what ES should be performed under the anesthetic setting of group F, because particular kind of risk management for anesthesia is always essential, and extensive training and experience are required.

Nevertheless, because ECT cannot be an effective therapy for drug-refractory and critically ill patients unless we can induce qualitatively effective seizures under the anesthesia protocols other than the anesthetic setting of group F, it should be considered sufficiently that their lives might not be saved in the end.

Fortunately, we have not yet encountered a serious complication resulting from the specific anesthetic setting of group F during ECT.

2.3 Comprehensive Monitoring and Management of Breathing, Sedation, and Circulation During ECT

Meticulous management of breathing, sedation, and circulation during ECT is critical for patient safety. We highlight the issues and dangers specific to anesthesia for ECT (Fig. 2.10).

2.3.1 Breathing Management and Monitoring

Of course, breathing management should be performed under proper sedation to relieve patient's anxiety and inhibit harmful autonomic reflexes during the procedure of anesthesia management for ECT.

Also, proper airway protection should be maintained to prevent aspiration of secretions into the lungs.

Besides, it is necessary to perform sufficient preoxygenation and to maintain enough oxygenation level by administering pure oxygen during anesthesia for ECT under monitoring by pulse oximetry.

On the other hand, hypoventilation at the time of ES reduces the chances of qualitatively effective seizure induction, so it is important to ensure proper ventilation without falling into hypoventilation [9].

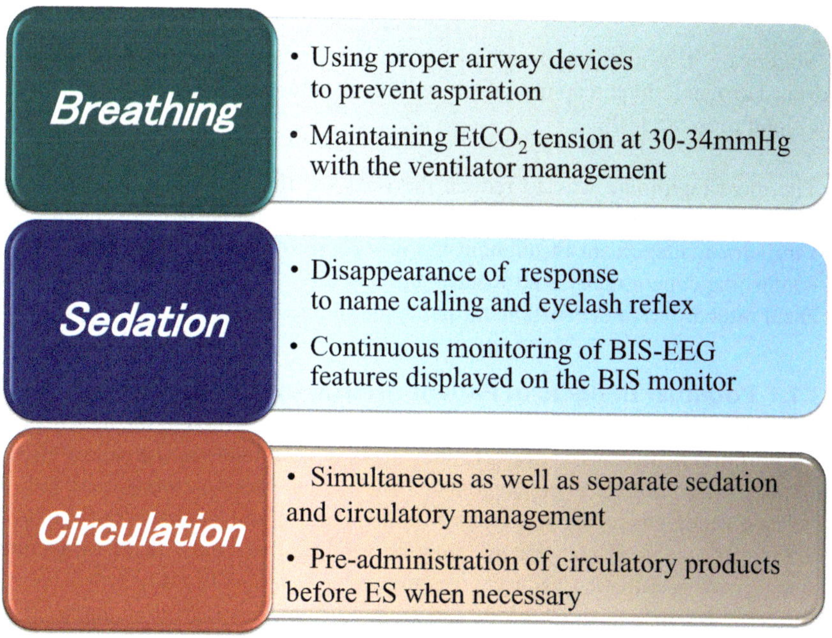

Fig. 2.10 Important matters of anesthesia management during ECT

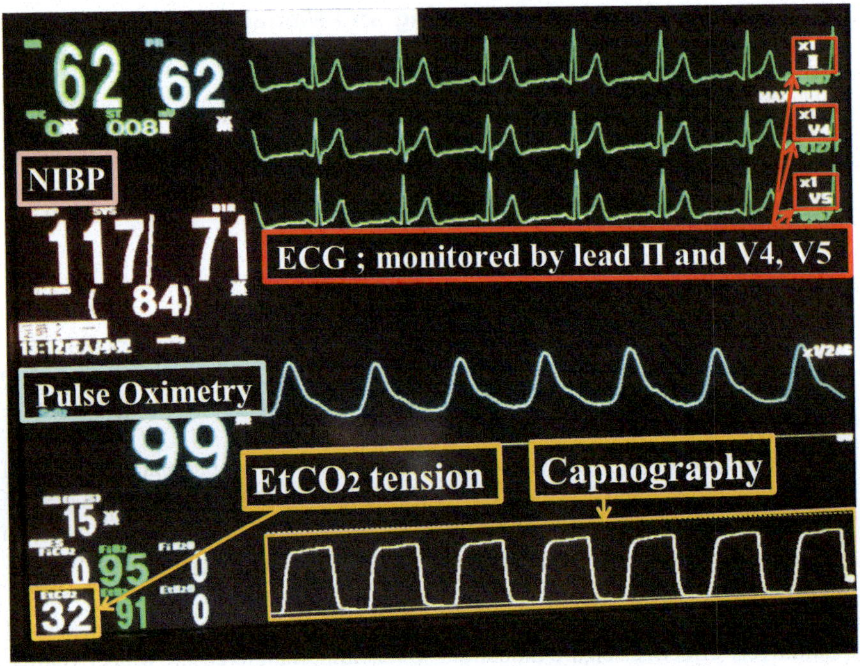

Fig. 2.11 $EtCO_2$ tension and capnography displayed on the monitor screen. Both $EtCO_2$ tension and capnography are displayed on the last line of the monitor screen

Moreover, it is also important to ensure proper ventilation following ES to prevent iatrogenic hypercapnia, which will result in a dangerous rise in heart rate and blood pressure [10].

- The most legitimate way to reduce the risks for those mentioned above is to confirm that $EtCO_2$ tension is maintained at the appropriate level with the ventilator management throughout the procedure of anesthesia for ECT, while confirming capnography after inserting proper airway devices (LMA or endotracheal intubation) under sufficient total depth of anesthesia (Figs. 2.11 and 2.12).

2.3.1.1 Potential Dangers of Patient Arousal by Respiratory Management Procedures

In the traditional anesthesia for ECT, anesthesia is often induced with a low effect-site concentration of a $GABA_A$ agonist. However, it does not reach the depth of anesthesia enough to suppress responses of the pharynx, and it is feared a vagovagal reflex may be induced and that we may be running the great risk of awakening patients, if we insert LMA or laryngoscopy under such conditions.

Probably because of this background respiratory management by manual mask ventilation is common during ECT. However, the noxious stimulus by manual mask-holding under a low effect-site concentration of $GABA_A$ agonist alone (i.e.,

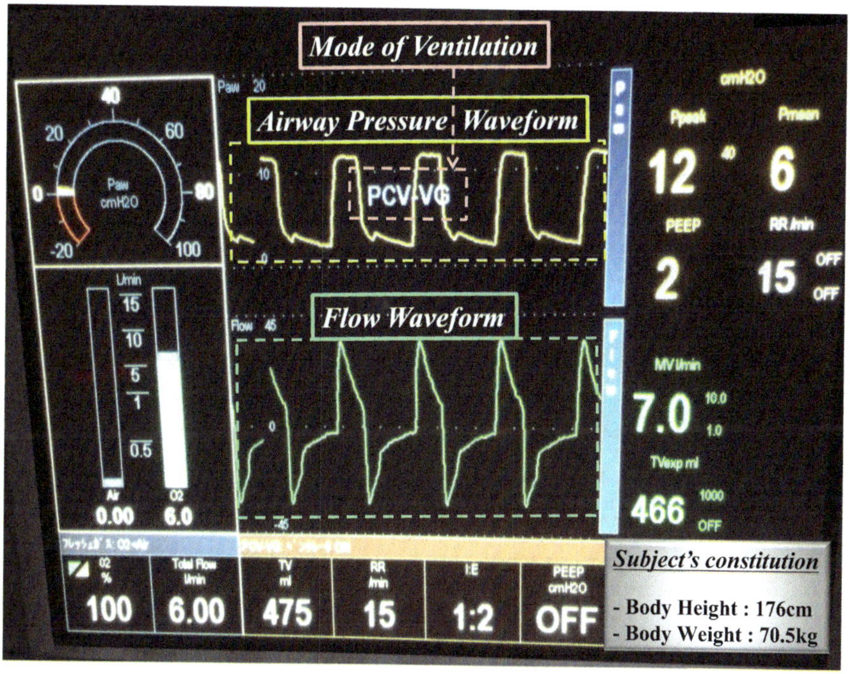

Fig. 2.12 Various information displayed on the anesthesia apparatus screen
Airway Pressure Waveform is displayed on the upper side of anesthesia apparatus screen. Flow Waveform is displayed on the lower side of anesthesia apparatus screen

without remifentanil) may also increase the risk of awakening the patient [11] (Fig. 2.13).

2.3.1.2 Potential Dangers of Aspiration Under Manual Mask Ventilation

Many potential patients for ECT are at greater risk of aspiration, such as subjects with swallowing difficulty due to stupor or catatonia. Such patients who are known or suspected to be repeating micro aspirations, it is often found that the secretions in pharynx have not been removed sufficiently by sucking-in treatment from oral cavity. When we auscultate the glottis area from the body surface, resistance sounds can be heard during inspiration and expiration. If manual mask ventilation is performed under such conditions, medicine-originated aspiration of secretions will occur as a matter of course [12].

In addition, patients at risk of gastroesophageal reflux due to coexisting illnesses, such as ileus, esophageal achalasia, or gastroparesis, are indicated for rapid sequence induction (RSI) in either case, and anesthesia induction of ECT should be performed as well by RSI in line with standard practices of anesthesia induction [13] (Fig. 2.14).

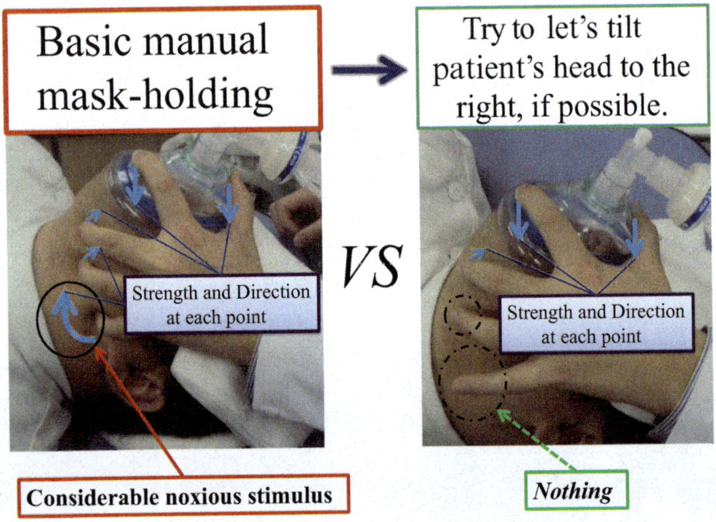

Fig. 2.13 Differences in noxious stimulus by the procedures of manual mask-holding
If BIS monitoring is used for the respiratory management under low effect-site concentration of only GABAA agonist, marked difference in noxious stimulus by the procedure of manual mask-holding will be plainly reflected in BIS-EEG features, which may consequently contribute to prevention of awareness during anesthesia

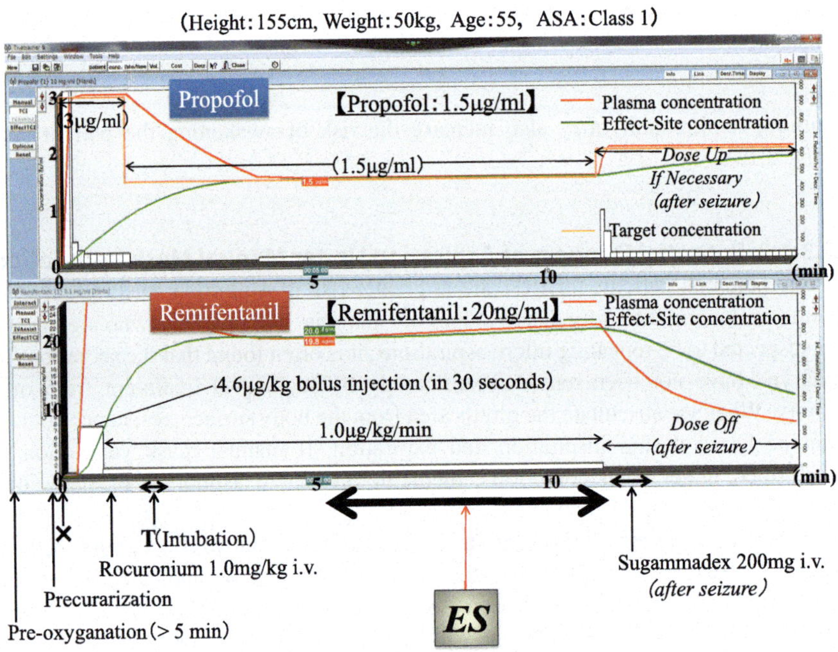

Fig. 2.14 Time course of anesthesia and electrical stimulation (Group A (RSI))

Moreover, when performing anesthesia management during ECT on subjects without these coexisting illnesses, it is still important to keep proper airway devices in place for unexpected airway events.

2.3.1.3 Problems in Accurate Evaluation of Seizure EEG When Resuming Manual Mask Ventilation

The parasympathetic nervous system is activated for a few seconds by ES, and the secretions from mucous membranes of the oral cavity and pharynx transiently increase. To prevent aspiration of these secretions, early sucking-in treatment is necessary. In contrast, it is not possible to predict seizure duration ahead of time, and patients are placed under breathless condition during it in case it lasts long; therefore, it is often necessary to resume manual mask ventilation before seizures cease. However, the procedure of opening the patient's mouth for sucking-in treatment before resuming manual mask ventilation causes sensors of seizure EEG and earth electrodes attached on patients to move at the same time (Fig. 2.6), and the baseline of seizure EEG results in the formation of inadequate swaying; thus, it leads to making accurate evaluation of seizure EEG, seizure end point, and postictal suppression difficult.

2.3.1.4 The Reliability of $EtCO_2$ Tension as an Indicator of Ventilatory Status

The correlation between $EtCO_2$ tension and $PaCO_2$ tension may be conducive to poorer reliability during respiratory management by manual mask ventilation due to individual differences in the anatomical dead space. Besides, patients with difficulties in mask ventilation also have a tendency to fall into hypoventilation, further decreasing the reliability of $EtCO_2$ tension as an indicator of ventilatory status.

For this reason, past studies involving respiratory management by manual mask ventilation during ECT have reported that continuous transcutaneous monitoring of pCO_2 ($TcPCO_2$) is a more useful indicator of ventilatory status [14].

2.3.1.5 Advantages of Our Practical Procedure of Respiratory Management

We recommend confirming that $EtCO_2$ tension is maintained at 30–34 mmHg with the ventilator management before attempting ES, while observing capnography after inserting proper airway devices (LMA or endotracheal intubation) under sufficient total depth of anesthesia. Doing so should obviate many of the problems mentioned (e.g., see Sects. 2.3.1.1, 2.3.1.2, 2.3.1.3, and 2.3.1.4).

On the other hand, laryngeal spasm and anaphylaxis are comparatively rare but serious airway and respiratory complications during ECT. It may not be difficult to determine the cause of laryngeal spasm and anaphylaxis by the difficulty in proper ventilation or by the patient's physical responses when respiratory management is being performed by manual mask ventilation. However, anesthesiologists' hands in a free condition (owing to the ventilator management with proper airway devices) among other things, as well as monitoring abnormal capnography, rise of peak pressure, and abnormal airway pressure waveform, are useful signals for prompt corrective action to prevent respiratory crises (Figs. 2.11 and 2.12).

2.3.1.6 Tricks and Traps of Our Practical Procedure of Respiratory Management

Several additional points should be emphasized when using our practical procedure of respiratory management during ECT.

First, precurarization is essential since high-dose remifentanil is administered intravenously when inducing anesthesia. Indeed, rigidity appears in some cases, particularly when inducing anesthesia with our anesthetic settings of groups E and F. However, in accordance with past studies [15], it is our experience that at the point when rigidity appears, consciousness is already not at a clear level according to patient's physical responses and BIS-EEG features. It is critical to never misjudge the appropriate time for administering muscle relaxant intravenously to ensure there are no troubles with intravenous lines and to avoid sending oxygen into the digestive tract by high-pressured manual mask ventilation. And though it is possible, if the patients have no respiratory or cardiac diseases which are likely to lead to hypoxia, to prevent a hypoxic state when ventilation with pure oxygen is begun after rigidity decreases or disappears, it definitely presupposes that sufficient pre-oxygenation has been performed ahead of time.

The risk of injuring teeth during ES should also be mentioned. As the electrical stimulus pad is attached close to the masseter muscle, vicious bites cannot be prevented for a few seconds during ES even when patients are under sufficient muscular relaxation. To prevent injuries to teeth, it is advisable to insert the teeth guard protector as far as possible and use LMA with a soft tube and bite block for exclusive use with ECT.

For further details of respiratory management during ECT, please refer to Chap. 4: Airway and respiratory management.

2.3.2 Sedation Management and Monitoring

As one of monitors to infer sedation levels during anesthesia management, BIS monitor is being frequently used today.

2.3.2.1 Essence of Proper BIS Monitoring

In BIS monitoring, sedation level is expressed numerically (between 0 and 100) by a BIS-value derived through multivariate analysis of EEG from a frontal lobe on one side by means of some kinds of parameters and coefficients. However, there are limitations to the BIS-value as it is only a statistical estimate over approximately 1 min, not a real-time measure of state of consciousness. On top of them, it is subject to the influence of sways of EEG-baseline and various sources of artifacts and noise. In addition, there is a possibility that it does not suite the parameters or multivariate analysis on calculating BIS-value, depending on effect-site concentration settings of propofol and remifentanil [16, 17].

For these reasons in order to make apposite use for the essence of BIS monitoring, it is quite important to observe BIS-EEG features carefully and continuously under conditions of enough signal quality index and no electromyogram noise (EMG noise) mixed in [18].

If BIS monitoring is used for anesthesia management during ECT, the electrical stimulus pad on the temple may interfere with BIS sensor No. 3. However, because BIS sensor NO. 3 is an earth electrode, we fit BIS sensor NOs. 1, 2, and 4 at the usual place and BIS sensor NO. 3 above outer eyebrow (Fig. 2.6). Although it may be more subject to noises from movements of the orbicularis oculi muscle and eyeball, conversely we have only to observe BIS-EEG features carefully while confirming there are none.

2.3.2.2 Unreliable BIS-Values Determined by Careful Observation of BIS-EEG Features Before Anesthesia Induction

When we observe the BIS monitor before anesthesia induction in ECT-subjects, we often find BIS-EEG features much EMG noise mixes in due to their too much strain in some cases or something like bursts of δ-waves due to their involuntary movement such as blinking in others.

Former cases are also observed before anesthesia in patients without psychiatric disorders and show high level of BIS-value, but because that does not reflect high relative β-ratio or γ-wave band activity on EEG but EMG noise as well, rating it as BIS-value before anesthesia induction is inappropriate in itself (Fig. 2.15a).

On the other hand, in the latter cases it is not rare that BIS-value shows 50 or less depending on the frequency of involuntary movement such as blinking or on how much EMG noise mixes in. However, when we observe BIS-EEG features carefully, EMG noise or β-waves can be stringently verified on greatly swaying EEG-baseline. In the same way, rating it as BIS-value before anesthesia induction is inappropriate in itself (Fig. 2.15b).

2.3.2.3 Assessment of Sedation Levels After Anesthesia Induction for ECT

Generally, it is extremely important to confirm disappearance of response to name calling and eyelash reflex when we judge loss of consciousness after anesthesia induction. However, some ECT-subjects will show the signs even before anesthesia induction due to stupor or catatonia.

Although it is confirmed of course ahead of time that abnormalities are not observed in head CT of such patients, β-waves are more frequently predominant in the basic EEG activity than in healthy people on the other hand.

When we are keeping on confirming BIS-EEG features, EMG noise is disappearing after anesthesia induction with the rise in effect-site concentrations of intravenous anesthetics, and it becomes possible to estimate BIS-EEG features more precisely which suggests that consciousness is not at a clear level.

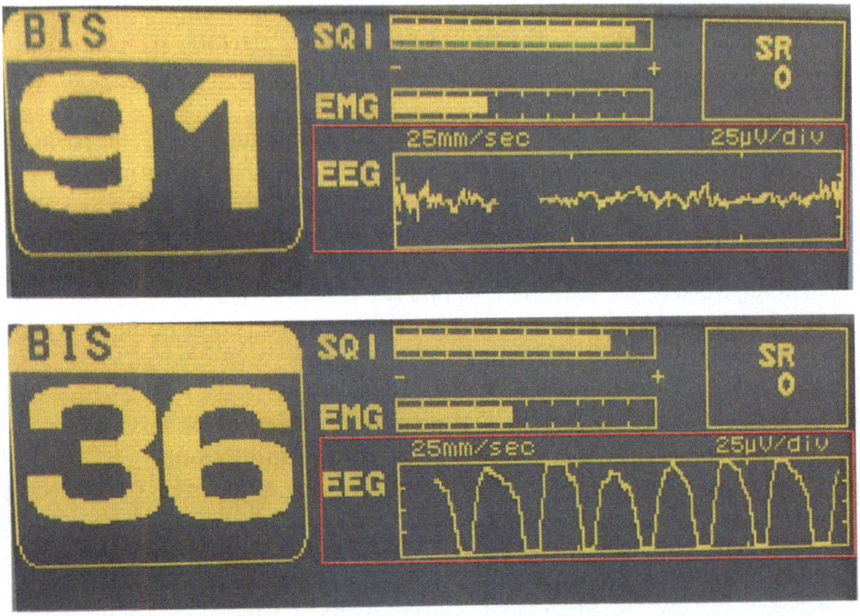

Fig. 2.15 Unreliable BIS-values determined by BIS-EEG features before anesthesia. (**a**) BIS-EEG features, much EMG noise mixes in, are shown in the upper side of this photogram. (**b**) EMG noise or β-waves on greatly swaying baseline are shown in the lower side of this photogram

2.3.2.4 Observed BIS-EEG Features After Anesthesia Induction

To put it concretely, β-waves are predominantly observed in BIS-EEG features derived from the frontal lobe of patients with no past brain injury or stroke, while awake and with eyes closed.

With lowering consciousness level after anesthesia induction, BIS-EEG features composed mainly of spindle waves are observed (Fig. 2.16a).

With further lowering consciousness level, both extremely low amplitude basic EEG activity and partially clustered slow waves (Fig. 2.16b) or bursts of δ-waves are observed in BIS-EEG features (Fig. 2.16c).

Using our anesthetic settings on ECT-subjects, these three kinds of BIS-EEG features are mostly observed during anesthesia induction as well.

When we apply our anesthetic settings of groups S, A', A, or B to young or middle-aged subjects, BIS-EEG features shown in Fig. 2.16a are relatively frequently observed.

On the other hand, when we apply our anesthetic settings of groups E or F to elderly subjects, bursts of δ-waves are observed in all cases as shown in Fig. 2.16c.

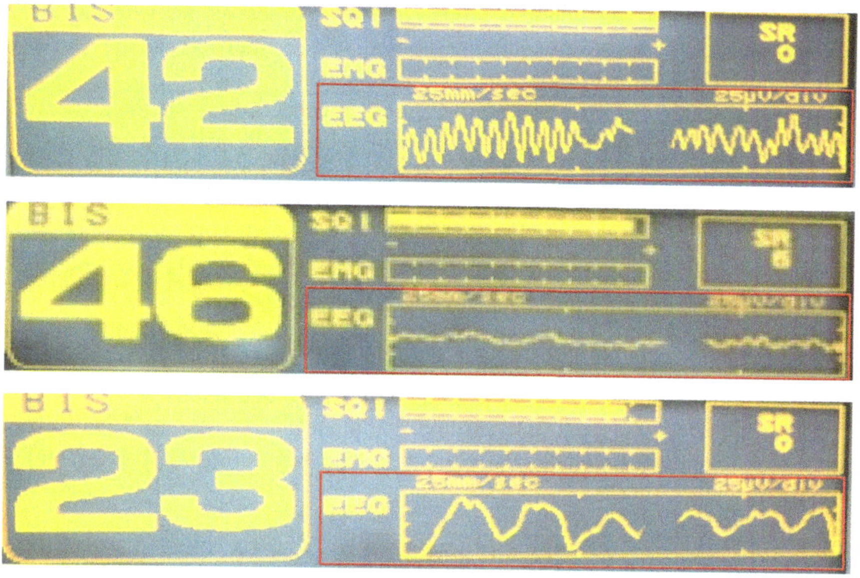

Fig. 2.16 BIS-EEG features after anesthesia induction. (**a**) EEG trace, mainly composed of spindle waves, is shown in the upper side of this photogram. (**b**) Both extremely low amplitude of basic EEG activity and partially clustered slow waves are shown in the middle side of this photogram. (**c**) Bursts of δ-waves are shown in the lower side of this photogram

2.3.2.5 Purpose of Continuous Visual Monitoring of BIS-EEG Features During Anesthesia Management for ECT

Continuous visual monitoring of BIS-EEG features is nothing but material for judging that the consciousness level is not clear at least. And we estimate patients' loss of consciousness comprehensively by confirming the disappearance of response to name calling and eyelash reflex and by the hemodynamic change in association with increased effect-site concentrations of intravenous anesthetics as well at the same time.

However, as it is another problem whether the anesthesia depth is sufficient to control hemodynamic changes before and after ES, it should be considered to administer circulatory products before ES, if necessary.

2.3.3 Circulatory Management and Monitoring

At the time of anesthesia induction, patients show various hemodynamic changes depending on the kind and concentration of intravenous anesthetics, general physical condition, and recent medication use, so anesthesiologists need to recognize ahead of time what types of circulatory management will be necessary according to each change.

Then, as the parasympathetic nervous system is temporarily activated for a few seconds by ES, harmful phenomena, such as severe bradycardia, are likely to appear and cardiac arrest can occur on rare occasions [19].

When qualitatively effective seizures are induced, the sympathetic nervous system is activated causing an acute rise in blood pressure and heart rate. In rare cases, complications such as fatal tachyarrhythmia may result [20].

As extreme hemodynamic changes are observed during ES, we perform 12-lead ECG and echocardiogram prior to ECT in all subjects to confirm whether they have various risk factors for these critical events, such as arrhythmia, ischemic ECG changes, cardiac valvular diseases, and depressed ejection fraction.

After comprehensive evaluation of cardiac function, we provide a full account of prospective risks for cardiac complications caused by ES and anesthesia during ECT and obtain informed consent from all patients or their relatives.

Unfortunately, cases of fatal cardiac complications during ECT have been reported, so circulatory management and monitoring during ECT is extremely important.

2.3.3.1 Monitoring of ECG and Required Procedure

Even when prior 12-lead ECG indicates no pre-existing cardiovascular complications, we continuously monitor the ECG before anesthesia induction.

If rare but severe abnormalities of ECG such as cardiac arrest or fatal tachyarrhythmia should be observed during ES, it is essential to practice rapidly what is needed to cope with them in a right manner, and to that end, we need to prepare circulatory products, cardioverter defibrillator, and trained staff in advance. Even in such cases, anesthesiologists' hands in a free condition should be a great advantage to perform prompter and more appropriate treatment of the crises.

Besides, to be alert for signs of myocardial ischemia, such as ST-segment abnormalities or inverted T-wave, we recommend that ECG should be monitored not only by lead II but also by leads V4 and V5 during ECT.

The upward-sloping type of transient ST-segment depression is relatively common on the ECG due to tachycardia after seizure induction, but it is not a pathological feature and is usually relieved within minutes after conclusion of the seizure (Fig. 2.17).

On the other hand, if horizontal or down-sloping type of ST-segment depression or inverted T wave is observed on the ECG probably due to relative myocardial ischemia associated with significantly increased cardiac output after seizure induction following ES, 12-lead ECG, echocardiogram, and a blood test, including determination of cardiac troponins, creatinine kinase (CK), and CK-MB, should be performed rapidly. And when it is not possible to suspend the scheduled ECT on the patient by necessity, it should be considered to administer nitric acid, β-blocker, and/or calcium-channel blocker concurrently at and after the next session.

Moreover, if ST-segment elevation caused by seizure induction following ES is observed on the ECG, complete examination for ischemic heart disease, including cardiac catheterization, must be performed immediately, and the scheduled ECT should be suspended or canceled in principle.

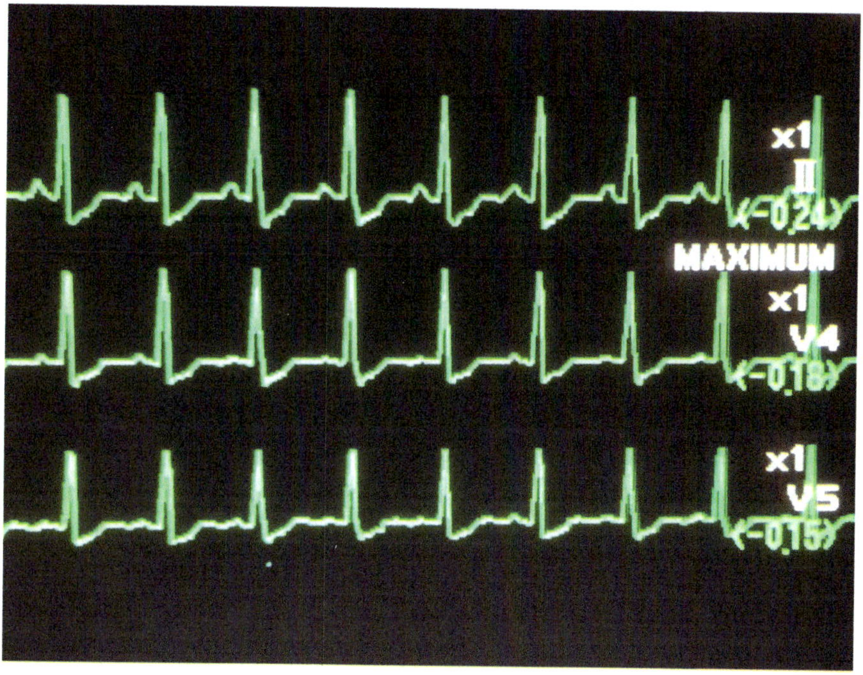

Fig. 2.17 Upward-sloping type of transient ST-segment depression due to tachycardia after seizure

2.3.3.2 Management and Monitoring of Blood Pressure and Heart Rate

In general, noninvasive arterial blood pressure and heart rate are monitored during ECT. However, continuous invasive hemodynamic monitoring should be considered for patients who have severe abnormalities of cardiac function according to medical history, current echocardiogram, and 12-lead ECG.

Regardless of regularly taken medications, when anesthesia is induced by our anesthetic settings of groups S, A', A, B, or C, we pay careful attention to the possibility of significant hypotension and bradycardia owing to the interactions among propofol, remifentanil, and psychotropic agents and consider administering 1–2 μg/kg phenylephrine or 10 μg/kg atropine intravenously if deemed necessary.

If the patient has regularly taken major tranquilizers, particularly phenothiazines, no matter which anesthesia protocol is used ($GABA_A$ agonist only or both $GABA_A$ agonist and remifentanil), we should pay more careful attention to possible significant hypotension owing to the interaction between intravenous anesthetics and major tranquilizers and consider to administer phenylephrine or noradrenaline intravenously if deemed necessary.

Conversely, when anesthesia is induced with only remifentanil as in our anesthetic setting of group F, a rise in blood pressure and heart rate is observed in nearly every instance, so it is necessary to administer calcium-channel blocker and β-blocker, such as nicardipine and landiolol, intravenously soon after anesthesia induction.

After seizure induction, the acute rise in both blood pressure and heart rate is caused by a catecholamine surge. As a matter of course, a certain level of hypertension and tachycardia should be permitted to prevent relative brain ischemia. Alternatively, strict control of blood pressure or heart rate is required for patients who have cerebral aneurysm or severe aortic valvular stenosis and hypertrophic obstructive cardiomyopathy.

Since extreme hemodynamic changes are often observed during the period from anesthesia induction to disappearance of seizure, it is desirable to have available adequate circulatory products, particularly just before ES, to respond to a variety of emergency situations.

Furthermore, we are required to recognize what sedation and circulatory management should be performed simultaneously as well as separately during anesthesia for ECT.

For further details of circulatory management during ECT, please refer to Chap. 5: Circulatory management especially blood pressure and heart rate.

2.4 Monitoring and Qualitative Evaluation of Seizure EEG and Postictal Suppression

ECT is a treatment strategy aimed at improving clinical symptoms through neurobiological basis resulting from generalized tonic-clonic seizure, which is induced by ES in whole brain, including temporal lobe, parietal lobe, occipital lobe, frontal lobe, and diencephalon [21, 22]. It has been reported that generalized tonic-clonic seizure EEG is observed more dominantly at the frontal lobe [23, 24]. It means that unless qualitatively effective seizure EEG derived from bilateral frontal lobes is at least observed after ES, we cannot induce generalized tonic-clonic seizure indeed, and rate as not therapeutically effective seizure EEG in other words.

Meanwhile, sufficient postictal suppression derived from bilateral frontal lobes is more frequently observed when seizure EEG after ES is qualitatively evaluated as valid. Indeed, it has been reported many times that sufficient postictal suppression is correlated with good response to treatment [25, 26].

2.4.1 Qualitative Evaluation of Seizure EEG

Seizure EEG after ES is qualitatively evaluated in clonic phase which appears following tonic phase (Fig. 2.18).

At that time, height of amplitude, regularity in amplitude and frequency, and right-to-left symmetry are counted as major rating items among others [26–28].

And for some time past, a methodology providing numerical scores of the properties of amplitude, regularity, and symmetry of seizure EEG (highest score: 6) has been reported [26, 29]. It would appear that scores 6 and 5 are regarded as

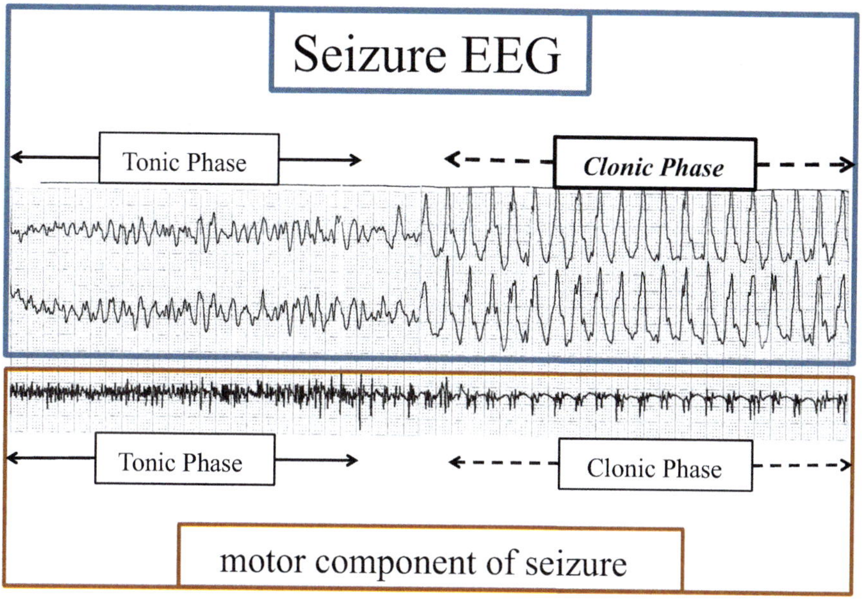

Fig. 2.18 Tonic and clonic phase of seizure

effective rating and scores 4 or less as not effective rating in this methodology (Fig. 2.19).

It is regretted, however, that the definitive value of amplitude or the objective indices of regularity and symmetry of seizure EEG remain open issues.

2.4.2 Qualitative Evaluation of Postictal Suppression

The criteria for qualitative evaluation of postictal suppression, focused on the appearance pattern of it, have been commonly known among psychiatrists, and a methodology for providing numerical scores of postictal suppression (highest score: 3) has been also reported [26, 29]. It would appear that scores 3 and 2 are regarded as effective rating (Fig. 2.20).

In our experience, sufficient postictal suppression (score 3 or 2) is observed in almost all cases when seizure EEG is qualitatively evaluated at score 6 or 5, and is more plainly reflected in BIS-EEG features as flat brain waves. When postictal suppression persists for more than 1 min, a BIS-value less than 10 is not rarely observed on the BIS monitor (Fig. 2.21).

However, the relationship between the duration of postictal suppression and recovery time to awakening or therapeutic response of patients remains less well defined.

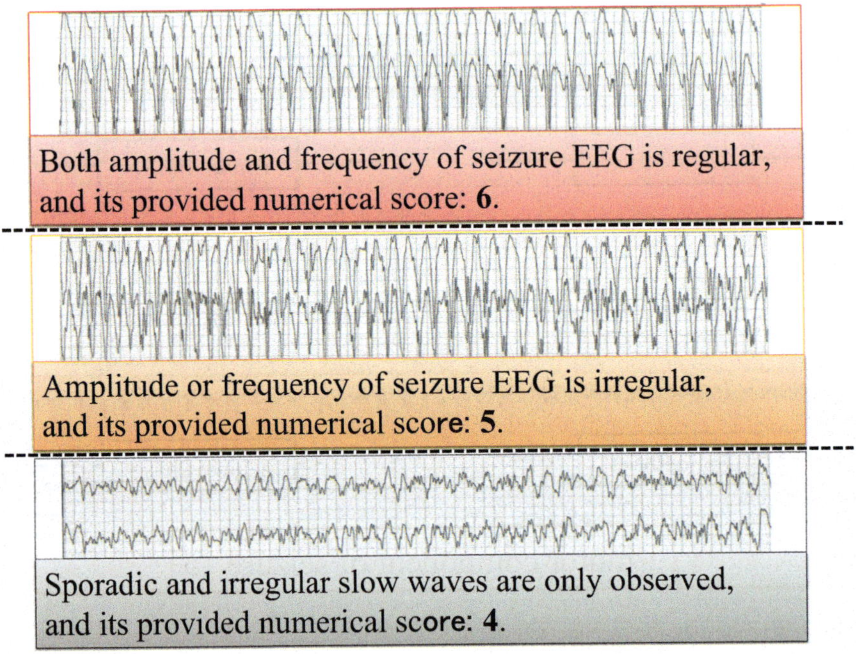

Fig. 2.19 Methodology for numerical scoring of seizure EEG properties

2.4.3 Common Fallacies About Seizure EEG Duration as an Indicator to Determine the Effectiveness of ECT

In many past studies, the seizure EEG duration has been reported as if it was an index of effectiveness. It is even probable that the seizure EEGs shown in Figs. 2.22 and 2.23 have been rated equally simply because they are of almost the same duration though they are of greatly different quality.

Today, the general idea that qualitative evaluation of seizure EEG and postictal suppression are both crucially important while seizure EEG duration is enough if only it lasts for more than 20–25 s is slowly gaining acceptance. At least we would like to emphasize here that the interpretation “the longer the duration, the more effective the seizure” is obviously wrong.

2.5 Concluding Remarks

In recent years, as the Thymatron System IV has come into wider use, monitoring and qualitative evaluation of seizures induced by ES has become possible. As a result, induction of qualitatively effective seizures under proper sedation, respiratory management, and cardiovascular stability is a stringent requirement for ECT. However, it is still difficult to meet all conditions in clinical practice. While there

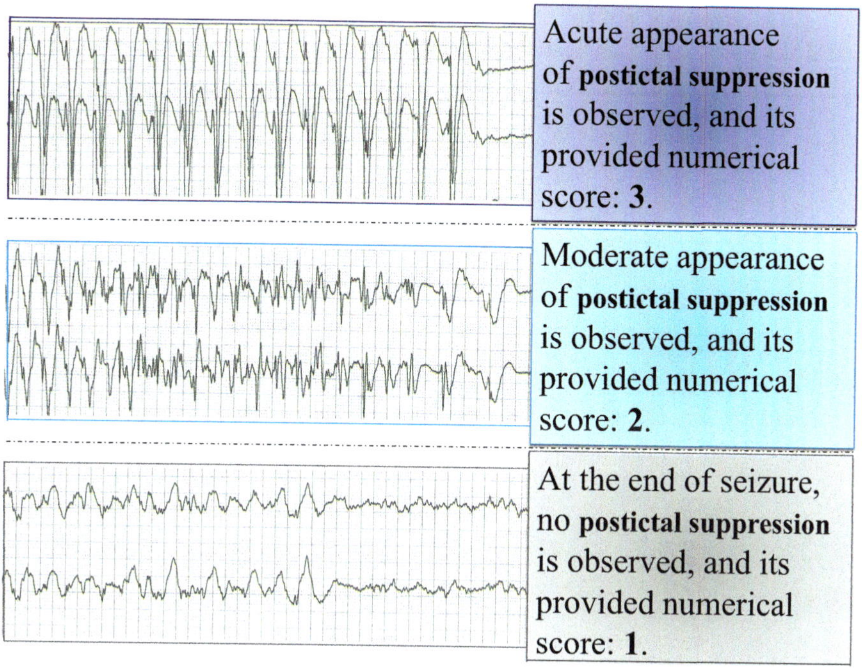

Fig. 2.20 Methodology for numerical scoring of postictal suppression pattern

are many factors making it difficult mainly because of differences in individual patients or resulting from anesthesia management, they are not known widely enough at present. Therefore, in addition to a full understanding of these problems, anesthesiologists must develop anesthesia procedures for ECT that possess methodological rationality. This task can be aided by the plethora of physiological monitoring devices and computer simulation software now available. Furthermore, sufficient knowledge and understanding of special characteristics and essence of those mentioned above is absolutely necessary.

While it goes without saying that physical remarks gained from patients in front of us as well as sharpened senses of anesthesiologists themselves are important, we believe that strict control of intravenous anesthetic concentrations with computer simulation software, strict monitoring of sedation, respiration, and hemodynamics, and readily available resources for crisis management will greatly contribute to safer and more effective use of ECT. Furthermore, every anesthesiologist should be made aware of more ratiocinative challenges and potential dangers associated with anesthesia for ECT.

ECT, with its extended applications on psychiatric disorders difficult to treat nowadays, continues to be an indispensable treatment as a unique life-saving measure.

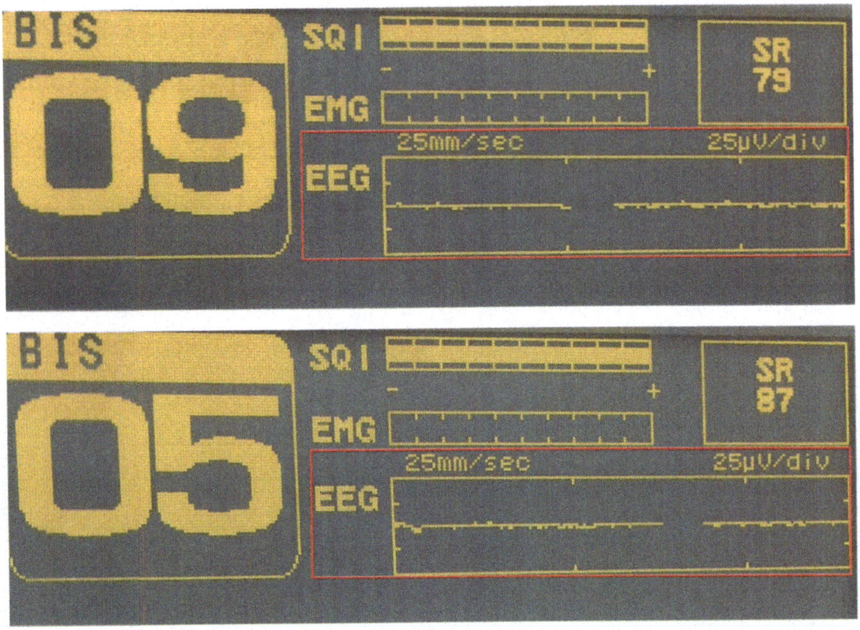

Fig. 2.21 Postictal suppression reflected in BIS monitor

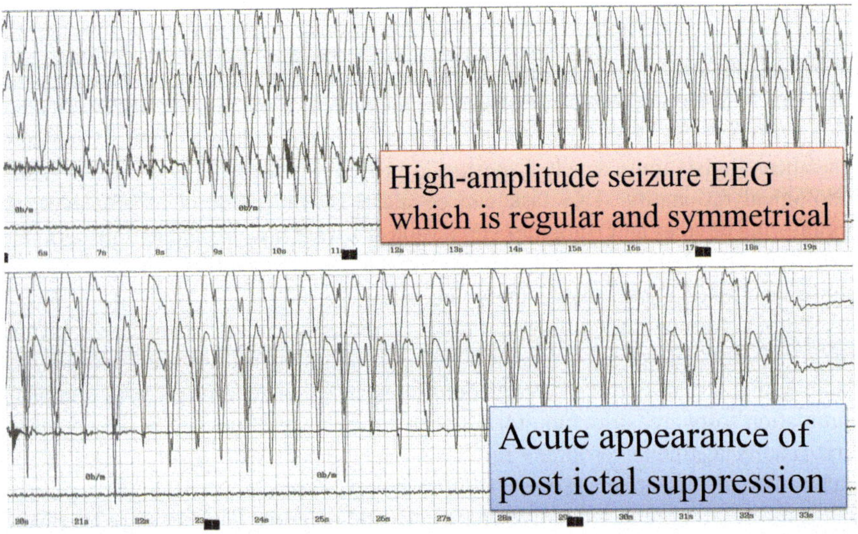

Fig. 2.22 EEG of a qualitatively effective seizure

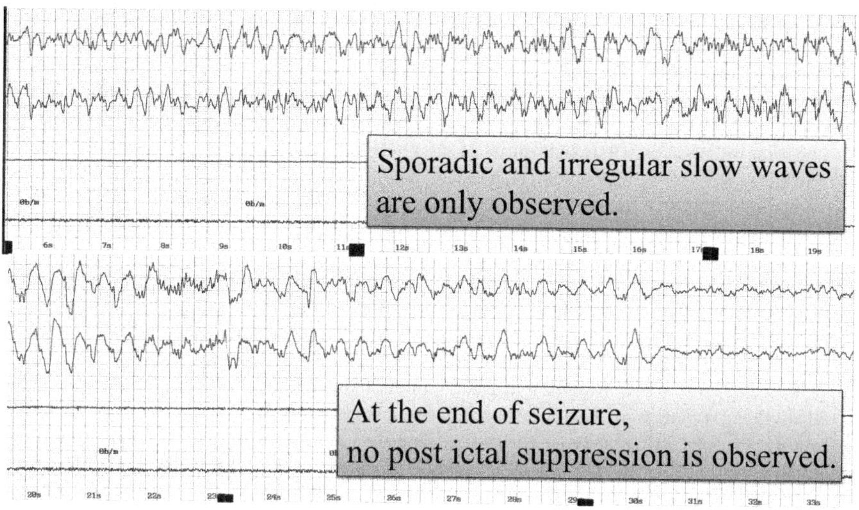

Fig. 2.23 EEG of a qualitatively invalid seizure

Eventually, improvements in monitors, computer simulations, anesthetic agents, and methods for the optimal use of all these tools will enhance the safety and therapeutic efficacy of ECT.

And it is expected to be of some help toward a methodological foundation as a basis of clinical studies related to mechanisms of action in ECT including functional neuroimaging study.

We will be happy if this article be helpful to all medical professionals engaged in clinical practice and research of ECT.

Acknowledgment We would like to thank every psychiatrist, internist, pharmacist, nurse, and all of the staff daily engaged in clinical support of ECT in Kouseikai Kusatsu Hospital.

References

1. Saito S. Anesthesia management for electroconvulsive therapy: hemodynamic and respiratory management. J Anesth. 2005;19(2):142–9.
2. Poulet E, Auriacombe M, Tignol J. Seizure threshold and ECT. Importance for good clinical practice of ECT. A review of literature. L'Encéphale. 2002;29(2):99–107.
3. Schüttler J, Ihmsen H. Population pharmacokinetics of propofol: a multicenter study. Anesthesiology. 2000;92(3):727–38.
4. Kern SE, Xie G, White JL, Egan TD. A response surface analysis of propofol–remifentanil pharmacodynamic interaction in volunteers. Anesthesiology. 2004;100(6):1373–81.
5. Johnson KB, Syroid ND, Gupta DK, Manyam SC, Egan TD, Huntington J et al. An evaluation of remifentanil propofol response surfaces for loss of responsiveness, loss of response to surrogates of painful stimuli and laryngoscopy in patients undergoing elective surgery. Anesth Analg. 2008;106(2):471–9, table of contents.

6. Koitabashi T, Johansen JW, Sebel PS. Remifentanil dose/electroencephalogram bispectral response during combined propofol/regional anesthesia. Anesth Analg. 2002;94(6):1530–3.
7. Kurita T, Morita K, Kazama T, Sato S. Influence of cardiac output on plasma propofol concentrations during constant infusion in swine. Anesthesiology. 2002;96(6):1498–503.
8. Frölich M, Dennis D, Shuster J, Melker R. Precision and bias of target controlled propofol infusion for sedation. Br J Anaesth. 2005;94(4):434–7.
9. Nishihara F, Ohkawa M, Hiraoka H, Yuki N, Saito S. Benefits of the laryngeal mask for airway management during electroconvulsive therapy. J ECT. 2003;19(4):211–6.
10. Saito S, Kadoi Y, Nihishara F, Aso C, Goto F. End-tidal carbon dioxide monitoring stabilized hemodynamic changes during ECT. J ECT. 2003;19(1):26–30.
11. Gajwani P, Muzina D, Gao K, Calabrese JR. Awareness under anesthesia during electroconvulsive therapy treatment. J ECT. 2006;22(2):158–9.
12. Kurnutala LN, Kamath S, Koyfman S, Yarmush J, SchianodiCola J. Aspiration during electroconvulsive therapy under general anesthesia. J ECT. 2013;29(4), e68.
13. Zibrak JD, Jensen WA, Bloomingdale K. Aspiration pneumonitis following electroconvulsive therapy in patients with gastroparesis. Biol Psychiatry. 1988;24(7):812–4.
14. Aksay SS, Bumb JM, Janke C, Hoyer C, Kranaster L, Sartorius A. New evidence for seizure quality improvement by hyperoxia and mild hypocapnia. J ECT. 2014;30(4):287–91.
15. Streisand JB, Bailey PL, LeMaire L, Ashburn MA, Tarver SD, Varvel J, et al. Fentanyl-induced rigidity and unconsciousness in human volunteers incidence, duration, and plasma concentrations. Anesthesiology. 1993;78(4):629–34.
16. Duarte LTD, Saraiva RÂ. When the bispectral index (bis) can give false results. Rev Bras Anestesiol. 2009;59(1):99–109.
17. Zanner R, Pilge S, Kochs E, Kreuzer M, Schneider G. Time delay of electroencephalogram index calculation: analysis of cerebral state, bispectral, and Narcotrend indices using perioperatively recorded electroencephalographic signals. Br J Anaesth. 2009;103(3):394–9.
18. Barnard J, Bennett C, Voss L, Sleigh J. Can anaesthetists be taught to interpret the effects of general anaesthesia on the electroencephalogram? Comparison of performance with the BIS and spectral entropy. Br J Anaesth. 2007;99(4):532–7.
19. Tang W-K, Ungvari GS. Asystole during electroconvulsive therapy: a case report. Aust N Z J Psychiatry. 2001;35(3):382–5.
20. Koga Y, Mishima Y, Momozaki M, Hiraki T, Ushijima K. A case of nonsustained ventricular tachycardia immediately following modified electroconvulsive therapy in a depressive patient. J Anesth. 2011;25(4):595–8.
21. Takano H, Motohashi N, Uema T, Ogawa K, Ohnishi T, Nishikawa M, et al. Changes in regional cerebral blood flow during acute electroconvulsive therapy in patients with depression Positron emission tomographic study. Br J Psychiatry. 2007;190(1):63–8.
22. Sackeim HA. The anticonvulsant hypothesis of the mechanisms of action of ECT: current status. J ECT. 1999;15(1):5–26.
23. Sakurai K, Takeda Y, Tanaka N, Kurita T, Shiraishi H, Takeuchi F, et al. Generalized spike-wave discharges involve a default mode network in patients with juvenile absence epilepsy: a MEG study. Epilepsy Res. 2010;89(2):176–84.
24. Holmes MD, Brown M, Tucker DM. Are "generalized" seizures truly generalized? Evidence of localized mesial frontal and frontopolar discharges in absence. Epilepsia. 2004;45(12):1568–79.
25. Edward C, Coffey M. The ictal EEG as a marker of adequate stimulus intensity with unilateral ECT. Neurosciences. 1995;7:295–303.
26. Nobler MS, Sackeim HA, Solomou M, Luber B, Devanand D, Prudic J. EEG manifestations during ECT: effects of electrode placement and stimulus intensity. Biol Psychiatry. 1993;34(5):321–30.
27. Motohashi N, Awata S, Isse K, Ueda S, Okubo Y, Okumura M, et al. Recommendation for ECT practice, Second edition. Psychiatria et neurologia Japonica. 2013;115(6):586–600.

28. Folkerts H. The ictal electroencephalogram as a marker for the efficacy of electroconvulsive therapy. Eur Arch Psychiatry Clin Neurosci. 1996;246(3):155–64.
29. McCall WV, Robinette GD, Hardesty D. Relationship of seizure morphology to the convulsive threshold. J ECT. 1996;12(3):147–51.

Selection of Anesthetics and Muscle Relaxants for Electroconvulsive Therapy

3

Yuji Kadoi

Abstract

Although the factors influencing seizure duration during electroconvulsive therapy (ECT) remain unknown, most anesthetic and hypotonic agents have some impact on seizure duration, ictal and postictal electrophysiological variables and the clinical efficacy of ECT. When a longer seizure duration is needed, etomidate, methohexital or a combination of small doses of a short-acting opiate with propofol are used.

The use of neuromuscular relaxants is essential to ensure patient safety during ECT. Succinylcholine is commonly used for its rapid onset and recovery. In patients with a history of neuroleptic malignant syndrome or neuromuscular diseases, a more promising method of muscle relaxation is to use rocuronium-sugammadex as an alternative to succinylcholine.

Keywords

Anesthetics • Seizure duration • Neuromuscular relaxants • Neuroleptic malignant syndrome

3.1 Anesthetic Agents for ECT

The ideal hypnotic agents for ECT should have a rapid onset and short duration of action, without the adverse effects of seizure activity induced by ECT. It is well known that selection of anesthetics and determination of the administered dose of the selected anesthetics are crucial in ECT management [1–5], because these factors have a potent impact on seizure induction during ECT. Although the

Y. Kadoi, MD, PhD (✉)
Department of Anesthesiology, Gunma University Hospital, 3-39-22 Showa-Machi, Maebashi, Gunma 371-8511, Japan
e-mail: kadoi@gunma-u.ac.jp

S. Saito (ed.), *Anesthesia Management for Electroconvulsive Therapy*,
DOI 10.1007/978-4-431-55717-3_3

Table 3.1 The effects of anesthetic agents on hemodynamics, cerebral blood flow and seizure duration

	Heart rate	Blood pressure	Cerebral blood flow	Seizure duration	Others
Methohexital	→/↑	↓	No change	→	
Thiopental	↑	↓	↓	↓	Histamine release
Propofol	→	↓	↓	↓	Most available
Diazepam	→/↑	↓	No change	↓↓	Long acting
Ketamine	↓	→/↑	↑	↓	
Etomidate	→/↑	↓	No change	↑	
Sevoflurane	↑	↓	↑	↓↓	

relationship between ECT seizure duration and its efficacy remains unclear, most of the available hypnotic agents shorten the seizure duration and increase seizure threshold. In addition, selected anesthetic agents could have differential effects on hemodynamic stability and emergence time (Table 3.1).

Physicians should be aware of the specific characteristics of the different hypnotic agents used for ECT, in regard to their effects on seizure duration, seizure threshold and systemic and cerebral hemodynamics. The success and safety of ECT depend on the appropriate choice of anesthetic drugs for the individual patient, which have to be chosen based on their individual concomitant medication and pre-existing diseases.

3.1.1 Methohexital

Currently, methohexital is the most recommended anesthetic for ECT [1–9]. Several guidelines [3, 4, 6] recommend methohexital administration at a dose ranging from 0.5 to 1.0 mg/kg for ECT induction. However, it has a dose-dependent anticonvulsive effect. Avramov et al. [7] compared the effects of methohexital, propofol and etomidate for ECT. Hypnosis was induced with an intravenous bolus injection of methohexital or propofol (both at doses of 0.75, 1.0 and 1.5 mg/kg), or etomidate (0.15, 0.2 and 0.3 mg/kg), administered over 10–15 s. The durations of EEG and motor seizures were longest after etomidate and shortest after propofol. Methohexital and propofol, at doses of 0.75, 1.0 and 1.5 mg/kg, produced dose-dependent decreases in motor and EEG seizure durations (Fig. 3.1), although the awakening times were similar, regardless of the hypnotic agent administered or its dose.

In an attempt to minimize the adverse effects of methohexital on shortening of ECT-induced seizures, Gurmarnik et al. [8] showed that divided doses of methohexital could minimize its adverse effects on seizure activity and improve outcomes after ECT.

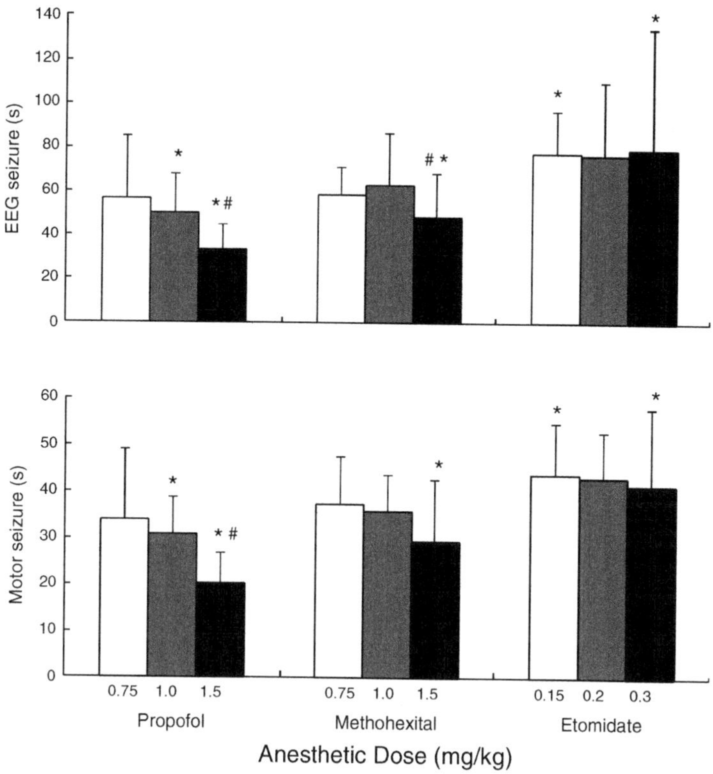

Fig. 3.1 Duration of motor and EEG seizures in patients receiving propofol, methohexital and etomidate (Avramov et al. [7])

3.1.2 Barbiturates

Barbiturates (thiopental and thiamylal) are alternatives to methohexital for anesthesia during ECT, although these drugs are associated with relatively short duration ECT seizures [10, 11]. In addition, more frequent arrhythmia was observed when using thiopental and thiamylal as compared to methohexital [9]. Mokriski et al. [9] showed that seizure duration was significantly prolonged by a mean of 5 s during methohexital anesthesia compared with thiopental sodium and thiamylal. The frequency of sinus bradycardia was lower with methohexital (8 %) compared with thiopental sodium (20 %) and thiamylal (20 %). The frequency of premature atrial contractions was lower with methohexital (43 %) compared with thiamylal (61 %), but not with thiopental sodium (57 %). The frequency of premature ventricular contractions was lower with methohexital (27 %) compared with thiopental sodium (44 %), but not with thiamylal (40 %). Atropine decreased the frequency of bradycardia (9 % vs. 24 %) and premature atrial contractions (47 % vs. 61 %) and increased the frequency of sinus tachycardia (88 % vs. 75 %). In our previous study series [1], we confirmed greater hemodynamic stability with

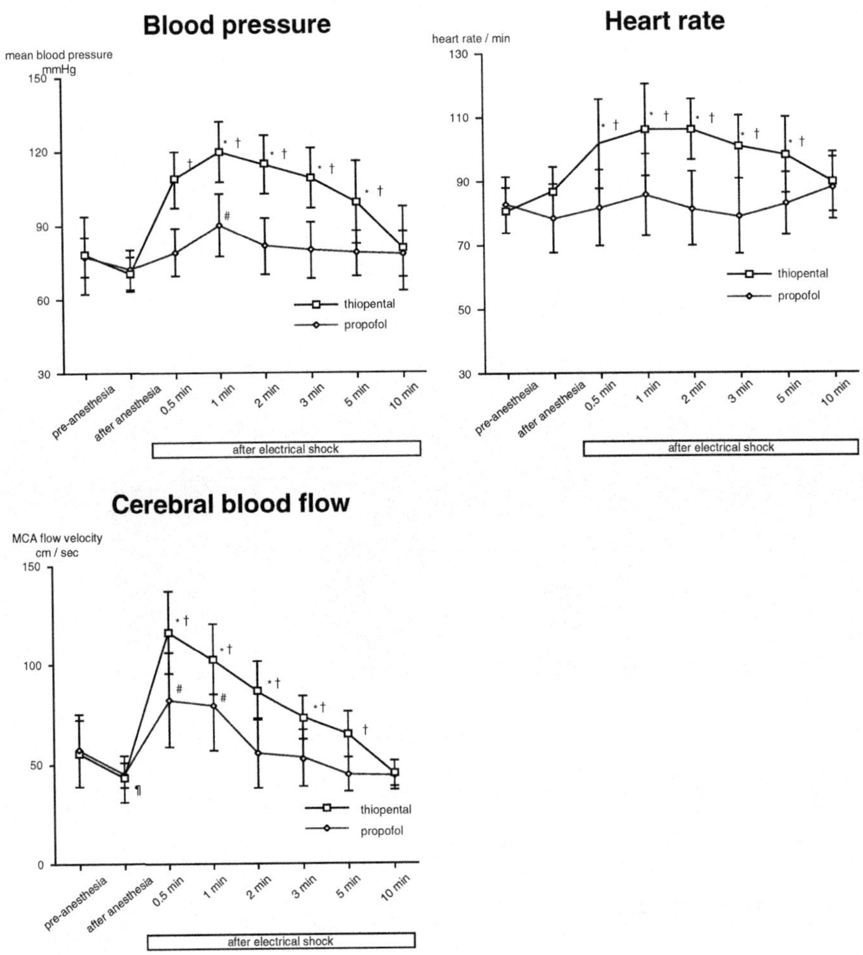

Fig. 3.2 Comparative effects of propofol (1.0 mg/kg) and thiopental (2.5 mg/kg) on blood pressure, heart rate and cerebral blood flow (Saito S et al. Anesth Analg 2000;91:1531–1536)

propofol than with barbiturates, because propofol has more profound cardiovascular dilatory effects compared with barbiturates (Fig. 3.2).

3.1.3 Propofol

The effects of propofol on ECT procedures have been examined by many researchers [12–24], who demonstrated that systemic and cerebrovascular hemodynamics are more stable under propofol as compared to barbiturate anesthesia. Although seizure duration under propofol anesthesia is shorter than that under barbiturate anesthesia, the psychiatric efficacy of ECT under both anesthetics is reportedly comparable [12–15]. Fear et al. [21] compared propofol and methohexital during ECT in patients with major depressive disorders (DSM-III-R criteria) in a prospective, randomized manner. They showed that although seizure duration was shorter with propofol, there was no difference in outcome, as measured by the Hamilton Depression Rating Scale and Beck Depression Inventory. Other studies by Fredman et al. [22, 23] showed that despite the shorter seizure duration observed in the propofol group as compared to the methohexital group, both hemodynamic stability and cognitive recovery were more favorable with propofol. Above all, it was concluded that doses of propofol <1.5 mg/kg are associated with a clinically acceptable duration of EEG seizure activity (>30 s) during ECT.

Interestingly, Imashuku et al. [16] reported the usefulness of a target control infusion (TCI) of propofol for the induction of ECT. However, with the TCI technique, the time required to achieve adequate hypnosis is relatively long. Hence, it is debatable whether a TCI of propofol is useful for ECT, as rapid induction of anesthesia is needed for ECT anesthesia.

3.1.4 Etomidate

Etomidate [25–29] is also used for ECT. Saffer et al. [28] and Trzepacz et al. [29] reported that etomidate ensured longer seizure duration when compared with both barbiturates and propofol. In contrast, more hemodynamic instability was often observed with etomidate as compared to both barbiturates and propofol. *However, the early cognitive recovery associated with etomidate may be delayed by post-ECT confusion*, and its use is associated with an increased incidence of emetic symptoms compared with propofol or methohexital.

3.1.5 Ketamine

Ketamine is also used for ECT and ensures longer seizure duration when compared to both barbiturates and propofol [30–35]. However, intracranial pressure elevation could be of concern when ketamine is used in ECT.

It is reported that ketamine, which is an n-methyl-d-aspartate (NMDA) receptor blocking agent, has antidepressant effects. Thus, it is plausible that the use of ketamine during ECT may enhance or accelerate ECT-induced antidepressant effects, compared with the use of propofol, methohexital or thiopental alone [31–35].

Yet, it remains controversial whether ketamine can enhance or accelerate the antidepressant effects of ECT [31–35]. Yoosefi et al. [35] demonstrated the efficacy of ketamine in regard to earlier improvement of depressive symptoms, longer seizure duration and better cognitive performance when compared to thiopental. In contrast, Järventausta et al. [33] showed that S-ketamine with propofol did not increase the effects of ECT in patients with treatment-resistant depression, and its use was associated with increased post-treatment disorientation and restlessness.

3.1.6 Benzodiazepines

It is well recognized that benzodiazepines can alter ECT-induced seizure threshold and duration [36–42]. Loimer et al. [38] compared the effects of midazolam and thiopental on ECT and reported that midazolam shortened the seizures to a duration that was not therapeutically desirable. Strömgren et al. [40] found in a retrospective study that the benzodiazepine group showed shorter seizure duration, more cases with insufficient seizure duration and a need for a greater number of treatments. They concluded that benzodiazepines should be administered with caution during ECT, as they can impair the efficacy of treatments and consequently prolong the treatment period. In contrast, Bush et al. [37] showed no adverse effects of lorazepam on ECT. Boylan et al. [36] reviewed that the average lorazepam, but not methohexital, dose in 48 h prior to ECT was likely to impact the increase in seizure threshold and is associated with decreased seizure duration.

Flumazenil, a GABA-A receptor antagonist, counteracts the effects of benzodiazepines, including sedation, memory loss, psychomotor impairment and respiratory depression. Many patients who receive ECT are benzodiazepine dependent or are anxious and require benzodiazepine drugs. It is possible that these benzodiazepine agents may diminish the therapeutic effectiveness of ECT. Krystal et al. [41] examined the dosing, safety and efficacy of pre-ECT administration of flumazenil, a competitive benzodiazepine antagonist, in patients receiving benzodiazepine medications and showed that although no differences in efficacy or seizure duration were found as a result of flumazenil administration, flumazenil offers the promise of safe and effective ECT in patients receiving benzodiazepine drugs. A recent study from Yi et al. [42] showed that flumazenil pretreatment of elderly ECT patients with declining seizure quality and inadequate clinical response may represent a novel strategy for managing such patients. However, further study is necessary to clarify the direct effect of the flumazenil/benzodiazepine combination or flumazenil alone on ECT-induced effects.

3.1.7 Sevoflurane

Use of sevoflurane has been demonstrated as being effective in stabilizing hemodynamics during ECT [43–48], although the associated time-consuming induction, relatively short seizure duration and requirement of an anesthesia machine make this technique impractical in most cases. Hodgson et al. [46] compared the effects of 8 % sevoflurane with propofol on ECT and found that the duration of seizure activity was longer with sevoflurane compared with propofol. Other studies from Rasmussen et al. [47], Toprak et al. [45] and Tanaka et al. [43] showed the usefulness of sevoflurane as an alternative anesthetic for ECT compared with propofol, methohexital or thiopental. In contrast, Calarge et al. [44] showed that when sevoflurane was used, seizure durations, recorded by observation and by EEG, were shorter by 10 and 23 s, respectively, compared with methohexital. In addition, they showed that methohexital allowed faster administration of ECT and discharge from the recovery room (3.8 vs. 6.2 min and 40.8 vs. 47.0 min, respectively). They concluded that sevoflurane might provide an alternative treatment option to methohexital, although with some limitations, including shortened seizure duration and potential side effects.

Sevoflurane is known to prolong the QT interval [48, 49]. Erdil et al. [48] showed prolongation of the QT interval when sevoflurane is used during ECT. Caution is, therefore, required when using sevoflurane during ECT because ECT-treated patients are often under antidepressant therapy, which also leads to prolongation of the QT interval [49].

3.1.8 Opiates

Opiates are not used alone as hypnotic agents during ECT anesthesia. However, many reports showed that combination of opiates with agents such as methohexital, thiopental or propofol improves short seizure duration or stabilizes systemic hemodynamics [50–54]. Dinwiddie et al. [50] reported that a combination of 25 μg/kg of alfentanil plus 20 mg of methohexital was associated with a 45 % increase in EEG duration. Beresford et al. [51] reported the successful treatment of two cases in which a combination of propofol-alfentanil anesthesia was used for ECT without any complications. Nguyen et al. [52] studied the effects of methohexitone and propofol with and without alfentanil on seizure duration and recovery in 24 patients. Each patient had four treatment sessions and received the following four IV regimens in random order: methohexitone 0.75 mg/kg, methohexitone 0.50 mg /kg and alfentanil 10 μg/kg, propofol 0.75 mg/kg, and propofol 0.50 mg/kg and alfentanil 10 μg/kg. Seizure durations were longest with methohexitone-alfentanil and shortest with propofol. Recovery time was shorter in patients receiving propofol compared with methohexitone-alfentanil and methohexitone alone. Alfentanil together with a reduced dose of methohexitone or propofol induced unconsciousness and increased seizure duration in patients undergoing ECT. Hence, they concluded that the combination of methohexitone with alfentanil was a good regimen for ECT, especially for patients who have short-duration seizures. Another study [53] reported the efficacy of remifentanil in preventing hyperdynamic responses induced by ECT. This study showed that mean motor seizure duration was significantly longer with methohexitone (0.5 mg/kg) plus remifentanil (1.0 μg/kg) (37.6+/−2.0 s) than with methohexitone (0.75 mg/kg) alone (27.1+/−11.5 s), and recovery time, time to spontaneous breathing and peak postictal changes in BP and HR were similar with both regimens. They concluded that a reduced dose of methohexitone combined with remifentanil allows a prolonged duration of motor seizures with ECT. In our opinion, low-dose methohexitone combined with a short-acting opioid is a reasonable alternative in elderly patients undergoing ECT and for other patients with short-duration seizures.

In contrast to alfentanil and remifentanil, when fentanyl (1.5 μg/kg IV) was administered with 0.75 mg/kg of methohexital, seizure duration was shortened [54]. Fentanyl also failed to attenuate the acute hemodynamic response to ECT. The increased seizure duration related to the short-acting opioid analgesics alfentanil and remifentanil appears to be associated with a reduction in IV anesthetic dose requirements. Therefore, in ECT patients with shorter-duration seizures, adjunctive use of a potent, rapid and short-acting opioid analgesic could be more beneficial.

3.1.9 Alternatives

Regardless of the type of anesthetics used in ECT, anesthetic dose is important in determining the adequacy of seizures induced by ECT. With most anesthetics, seizure duration becomes shorter with an increase in anesthetic dose [54]. Some articles have described hypnosis as satisfactory for ECT [22, 55], because electrical stimulation itself has potent neuro-suppressive actions and induces retrograde amnesia in the postictal phase. The minimum anesthesia depth required at the time of muscle relaxation and prior to electrical stimulation is probably unconsciousness, since muscle relaxation under an extremely shallow anesthetic state is considered unethical. Recently, bispectral index has been widely used to monitor anesthetic depth [56, 57]. However, several reports have described the value as unreliable under certain conditions, including after electrically induced seizures [58–61]. Some patients are completely awake even at a very low BIS value after ECT. However, consciousness prior to electrical stimulation can be monitored by this system. Nishihara et al. [60] and White et al. [61] demonstrated that the index can be used to titrate the dose of propofol or methohexital in ECT. By referring to the BIS value immediately before electrical stimulation, operators might be able to control seizure duration to some extent. However, this approach is only applicable provided propofol or methohexital is used consistently throughout ECT sessions. Lemmens et al. [62] reported that when different types of anesthetics are used, comparison across anesthetics cannot be obtained by this system.

3.1.10 Summary

Recent psychiatric studies demonstrated that therapeutic efficacy is not necessarily related to seizure duration [62–64]. Only abortive or extremely short seizures (of less than 15 s) are of concern [63, 64]. Physicians should weigh the risks and benefits of anesthetics and anti-hypertensive regimens in their ECT management, especially for patients with cardiac or vascular complications, when selecting the anesthetic agents.

3.2 Muscle Relaxants for ECT

Without the use of any neuromuscular relaxants, patients treated with ECT will require vigorous physical restraint and will have severe muscle pain after the ECT. In addition, bone fractures have been also reported with performance of ECT without any neuromuscular relaxants [65, 66]. Consequently, the use of neuromuscular relaxants is needed to minimize the convulsive motor activity, in order to prevent bone fractures and physical injury during the seizure, which is important in patients with osteoporosis or spinal injury.

The ideal characteristics of muscle relaxants for ECT are [65] ability to reduce the motor activity induced by ECT to avoid injury, [66] no adverse effects on seizure activity and [67] rapid recovery of spontaneous breathing without residual paralysis.

Although succinylcholine (suxamethonium) causes a variety of adverse effects, such as elevation of internal gastric pressure, myalgia, hyperkalemia and possible association of malignant hyperthermia, it is the most useful and commonly available neuromuscular relaxant agent, because of its short duration of action and rapid recovery [67].

3.2.1 Succinylcholine (Suxamethonium)

Succinylcholine, 0.5–1 mg/kg, is commonly used in ECT because of its short duration of action [1, 67]. Although several ultra-short-acting nondepolarizing muscle relaxants have been developed, none of these have a shorter duration of action than succinylcholine [1, 67]. Further, the potent muscle contraction impulse during electrically induced seizures may not be satisfactorily inhibited by nondepolarizing agents [1]. Muscle relaxation can be temporarily reversed by electrical stimulation. Therefore, even now, the use of nondepolarizing muscle relaxants is limited to patients suspected of having malignant hyperthermia [1, 67]. The ECT guidelines of the Royal College of Psychiatrists recommend a 0.5 mg/kg dose of succinylcholine for ECT modification. Murali et al. [68] compared the effects of the dose recommended by the Royal College of Psychiatrists (0.5 mg/kg) and a larger dose (1.0 mg/kg) on ECT procedures and showed that although a small delay in recovery from the respiratory paralysis occurred, the larger dose (1.0 mg/kg) was more effective in modifying the peripheral convulsion. Recently, Matsumoto et al. [69] examined the appropriate interval between succinylcholine (1.0 mg/kg) administration and electrical stimulation using a noninvasive impedance cardiac monitor and showed that the onset of muscular relaxation was related to cardiac output before succinylcholine administration (Fig. 3.3) [69]. This study indicated that the effect of a muscle relaxant should be confirmed by neuromuscular monitoring before electrical stimulation.

Williams et al. [70] reported the unsuspected prolongation of recovery from succinylcholine due to pseudocholinesterase deficiency in a patient undergoing ECT. Physicians must be aware of alternative muscle relaxants to succinylcholine (see section on rocuronium), in case of contraindications to succinylcholine, such as

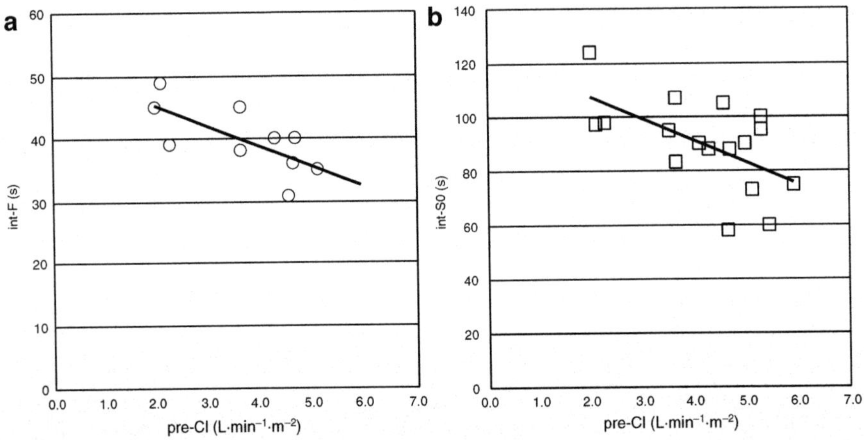

Fig. 3.3 Relationship between cardiac output and the onset of succinylcholine effects in ECT patients (Matsumoto et al. [69])

neuromuscular diseases, hyperkalemia [71] and a history of susceptibility to malignant hyperthermia (MH).

3.2.2 Mivacurium

Mivacurium, a relatively short-acting nondepolarizing neuromuscular agent, has been used as an alternative to succinylcholine during ECT [72–74]. Cheam et al. [74] compared the efficacy of mivacurium (0.08 mg/kg) with that of succinylcholine (0.5 mg/kg) in modifying seizure activity in 16 patients and showed that although mivacurium was unsatisfactory in eight cases compared with two cases after succinylcholine, clinical assessments of recovery from both relaxants were similar. Fredman et al. [75] performed a dose-effect study of mivacurium (0.12–0.2 mg/kg) in a patient with a history of neuroleptic malignant syndrome and showed that only 0.2 mg/kg of mivacurium (a full intubating dose) was associated with effective muscle relaxation during ECT. Gitlin et al. [76] also found that 0.15–0.25 mg/kg of mivacurium was needed to produce muscle relaxation for ECT in patients with myasthenia gravis.

Mivacurium is metabolized by pseudocholinesterase, so that caution must be exercised in patients with pseudocholinesterase deficiency. In addition, since mivacurium can induce a massive histamine release, hypotension after the administration of mivacurium should be watched for.

3.2.3 Atracurium and Rapacuronium

Lui et al. [77] examined the effects of two different doses (0.3 or 0.5 mg/kg) of atracurium on modification of tonic-clonic convulsions in ECT. They showed that patients receiving 0.5 mg/kg of atracurium had significantly fewer ECT-induced moderate and vigorous convulsions as compared to patients receiving 0.3 mg/kg of atracurium (moderate: 16.7 % vs. 78.4 %, vigorous: 0 % vs. 8.3 %). They suggested that 0.3 mg/kg of atracurium may be useful when one needs to ascertain the occurrence of ECT-induced seizures, as indicated by minimum peripheral muscle activity at the time of EEG activity indicative of seizures. Hickey et al. [78] compared the effects of succinylcholine (2–5 mg) and atracurium (10–15 mg) in a patient with atypical plasma cholinesterase and showed that the onset of action was 6 min for both relaxants, and time to 90 % recovery of the first twitch was 20 min for succinylcholine and 16 min for the atracurium-edrophonium combination. They concluded that the use of atracurium in these patients does not offer marked advantages over small doses of succinylcholine.

Kadar et al. [79] reported the use of rapacuronium for ECT in a patient with a family history of malignant hyperthermia. Rapacuronium was found to produce more rapid spontaneous recovery of neuromuscular function than other neuromuscular agents of the aminosteroid class. However, since rapacuronium can induce severe (even life-threatening) bronchospasm, it should not be used for muscle relaxation for ECT.

3.2.4 Vecuronium

Vecuronium is used for pretreatment in patients with severe succinylcholine-induced myalgia [80]. Sakamoto et al. [24] reported that propofol and vecuronium were safely used in ECT without complications in a patient with a history of neuroleptic malignant syndrome. Subsequently, Setoyama et al. [81] used 0.01 mg/kg of vecuronium, followed by another dose of 0.1 mg/kg in patients with neuroleptic malignant syndrome, and found a prolonged anesthesia time (30 vs. 19 min) in comparison with patients who received succinylcholine.

3.2.5 Rocuronium

Rocuronium, also a relatively short-acting nondepolarizing neuromuscular agent, has been used as an alternative to succinylcholine during ECT [82, 83]. Turkkal et al. [82] reported that although the time to the first spontaneous breath was longer in the rocuronium group than in the succinylcholine group, no significant differences were detected between the two groups in terms of eye opening, head lift or tongue depressor testing. However, the dosage of rocuronium used in the study of Turkkal et al. [82] was relatively small (0.3 mg/kg), which is thought to be inadequate for muscle paralysis.

Sugammadex has recently been introduced as a fast-acting, selective relaxant-binding agent that was specifically designed to rapidly reverse rocuronium-induced neuromuscular blockade. Lee et al. [84] reported that reversal of profound, high-dose rocuronium-induced neuromuscular block with 16 mg/kg sugammadex was significantly faster than spontaneous recovery from succinylcholine. Recently, there are some reports showing the efficacy of rocuronium-sugammadex as an alternative to succinylcholine for muscle relaxation during ECT [85–87]. Hoshi et al. [85] first described the usefulness of rocuronium (0.6 mg/kg)-sugammadex (16 mg/kg) as an alternative to succinylcholine. Subsequently, Kadoi et al. [86] compared the recovery times from rocuronium (0.6 mg/kg)-induced muscle relaxation after reversal with three different doses of sugammadex, with recovery from succinylcholine, and showed that 8 mg/kg of sugammadex produces equally rapid recovery from rocuronium-induced muscular relaxation compared with spontaneous recovery from 1 mg/kg succinylcholine (Tables 3.2 and 3.3).

3.2.6 Muscle Relaxants for Patients with a History of Neuroleptic Malignant Syndrome or Neuromuscular Diseases

Patients with a history of neuroleptic malignant syndrome (NMS) have been safely managed with succinylcholine chloride according to many case reports. Several reviews [88–90] and a case report [91] showed that succinylcholine can be safely used for ECT in these patients. However, when hyperthermic episodes cannot be conclusively diagnosed as NMS, avoiding the use of succinylcholine is recommended [92]. In patients with either NMS or MH, body temperature should

Table 3.2 The recovery time to T 1 of 10 % or 90 % in three differential doses of sugammadex (Time from commencement of administration of neuromuscular blocking agents to T1 of zero, and the time from commencement of administration of neuromuscular blocking agents to recovery of T1 to 10 and 90 %)

	T1 0 % (sec)	Recovery time to T1 of 10 % (sec)	Recovery time to T1 of 90 % (sec)
SCC	109 ± 28	310 ± 38	429 ± 65
Ro 0.6 mg/kg	123 ± 28		
	P value 0.13		
Sug 16 mg/kg		280 ± 54	387 ± 63*
Sug 8 mg/kg		324 ± 68	462 ± 66
Sug 4 mg/kg		407 ± 74*	563 ± 45*#

Ro Rocuronium, *Sug* Sugammadex, *SCC* Succinylcholine
*$p < 0.05$ compared with SCC
#$p < 0.05$ compared with Sug 16 mg/kg

Table 3.3 Seizure duration and time to first spontaneous breath

	Seizure duration (sec)	Time to first spontaneous breath (sec)
SCC	36 ± 6	273 ± 43
Sug 16 mg/kg	38 ± 4	233 ± 53*
Sug 8 mg/kg	40 ± 7	267 ± 69
Sug 4 mg/kg	39 ± 5	360 ± 59*#

Ro Rocuronium, *Sug* Sugammadex, *SCC* Succinylcholine
*$p < 0.05$ compared with SCC
#$p < 0.05$ compared with Sug 16 mg/kg

be carefully monitored, and therapeutic drugs and cooling strategies should be immediately available for use throughout the therapy schedule. Possibly, the most promising method of muscle relaxation in patients with a history of neuroleptic malignant syndrome or neuromuscular diseases is to use rocuronium-sugammadex [85, 86, 93]. Kadoi et al. [86] showed that rocuronium (0.6 mg/kg)-sugammadex (8 mg/kg) had equipotent efficacy as succinylcholine (1.0 mg/kg) in terms of both induction time of neuromuscular effects and recovery from neuromuscular effects, although at a higher cost.

3.2.7 Summary

Neuromuscular relaxants are needed to ensure patient safety during ECT. The ideal neuromuscular relaxant should have rapid onset of neuromuscular blocking effects and rapid recovery from the effects, because of which succinylcholine is commonly used. However, under specific conditions, such as a history of neuroleptic malignant syndrome or neuromuscular diseases, the most promising method of muscle relaxation seems to be the use of rocuronium-sugammadex as an alternative to succinylcholine.

References

1. Kadoi Y, Saito S. Anesthetic considerations for electroconvulsive therapy – especially hemodynamic and respiratory management. Curr Psychiatr R. 2009;5:276–86.
2. Ding Z, White PF. Anesthesia for electroconvulsive therapy. Anesth Analg. 2002;94:1351–64.
3. Rasmussen K. The practice of electroconvulsive therapy: recommendations for treatment, training, and privileging (second edition). J ECT. 2002;18:58–9.
4. Wagner KJ, Möllenberg O, Rentrop M, Werner C, Kochs EF. Guide to anaesthetic selection for electroconvulsive therapy. CNS Drugs. 2005;19:745–58.
5. Hooten WM, Rasmussen Jr KG. Effects of general anesthetic agents in adults receiving electroconvulsive therapy: a systematic review. J ECT. 2008;24:208–23.
6. Cook A, Stevenson G, Scott AI. A survey of methohexitone use by anesthetists in the clinical practice of ECT in Edinburgh. J ECT. 2000;16:350–5.
7. Avramov MN, Husain MM, White PF. The comparative effects of methohexital, propofol, and etomidate for electroconvulsive therapy. Anesth Analg. 1995;81:596–602.
8. Gurmarnik S, Young R, Alesker E. Divided doses of methohexitone improves ECT outcome. Can J Anaesth. 1996;43:535.
9. Mokriski BK, Nagle SE, Papuchis GC, Cohen SM, Waxman GJ. Electroconvulsive therapy-induced cardiac arrhythmias during anesthesia with methohexital, thiamylal, or thiopental sodium. J Clin Anesth. 1992;4:208–12.
10. Stromgren LS, Dahl J, Fjeldborg N, Thomsen A. Factors influencing seizure duration and number of seizures applied in unilateral electroconvulsive therapy. Anaesthetics and benzodiazepines. Acta Psychiatr Scand. 1980;62:158–65.
11. Boey WK, Lai FO. Comparison of propofol and thiopentone as anaesthetic agents for electroconvulsive therapy. Anaesthesia. 1990;45:623–8.
12. Geretsegger C, Nickel M, Judendorfer B, Rochowanski E, Novak E, Aichhorn W. Propofol and methohexital as anesthetic agents for electroconvulsive therapy: a randomized, double-

blind comparison of electroconvulsive therapy seizure quality, therapeutic efficacy, and cognitive performance. J ECT. 2007;23:239–43.
13. Geretsegger C, Rochowanski E, Kartnig C, Unterrainer AF. Propofol and methohexital as anesthetic agents for electroconvulsive therapy (ECT): a comparison of seizure-quality measures and vital signs. J ECT. 1998;14:28–35.
14. Mårtensson B, Bartfai A, Hallén B, Hellström C, Junthé T, Olander M. A comparison of propofol and methohexital as anesthetic agents for ECT: effects on seizure duration, therapeutic outcome, and memory. Biol Psychiatry. 1994;35:179–89.
15. Rasmussen KG. Propofol for ECT anesthesia a review of the literature. J ECT. 2014;30:210–5.
16. Imashuku Y, Kitagawa H, Kojima A, Ishikawa Y, Kuzukawa A, Nosaka S. Anesthetic management for electroconvulsive therapy using target-controlled infusion of propofol. Masui. 2008;57:889–91. Japanese.
17. Sakamoto A, Hoshino T, Suzuki N, Suzuki H, Kimura M, Ogawa R. Effects of propofol anesthesia on cognitive recovery of patients undergoing electroconvulsive therapy. Psychiatry Clin Neurosci. 1999;53:655–60.
18. Kirkby KC, Beckett WG, Matters RM, King TE. Comparison of propofol and methohexitone in anaesthesia for ECT: effect on seizure duration and outcome. Aust N Z J Psychiatry. 1995;29:299–303.
19. Matters RM, Beckett WG, Kirkby KC, King TE. Recovery after electroconvulsive therapy: comparison of propofol with methohexitone anaesthesia. Br J Anaesth. 1995;75:297–300.
20. Malsch E, Gratz I, Mani S, Backup C, Levy S, Allen E. Efficacy of electroconvulsive therapy after propofol and methohexital anesthesia. Convuls Ther. 1994;10:212–9.
21. Fear CF, Littlejohns CS, Rouse E, McQuail P. Propofol anaesthesia in electroconvulsive therapy. Reduced seizure duration may not be relevant. Br J Psychiatry. 1994;165:506–9.
22. Fredman B, D'Etienne J, Smith I, Husain MM, White PF. Anesthesia for electroconvulsive therapy: effects of propofol and methohexital on seizure activity and recovery. Anesth Analg. 1994;79:75–9.
23. Fredman B, Husain MM, White PF. Anaesthesia for electroconvulsive therapy: use of propofol revisited. Eur J Anaesthesiol. 1994;11:423–5.
24. Sakamoto A, Hoshino T, Suzuki H, Kimura M, Ogawa R. Repeated propofol anesthesia for a patient with a history of neuroleptic malignant syndrome. Nihon Ika Daigaku Zasshi. 1999;66:262–5.
25. Tan HL, Lee CY. Comparison between the effects of propofol and etomidate on motor and electroencephalogram seizure duration during electroconvulsive therapy. Anaesth Intensive Care. 2009;37:807–14.
26. Gazdag G, Kocsis N, Tolna J, Iványi Z. Etomidate versus propofol for electroconvulsive therapy in patients with schizophrenia. J ECT. 2004;20:225–9.
27. Gábor G, Judit T, Zsolt I. Comparison of propofol and etomidate regarding impact on seizure threshold during electroconvulsive therapy in patients with schizophrenia. Neuropsychopharmacol Hung. 2007;9:125–30.
28. Saffer S, Berk M. Anesthetic induction for ECT with etomidate is associated with longer seizure duration than thiopentone. J ECT. 1998;14:89–93.
29. Trzepacz PT, Weniger FC, Greenhouse J. Etomidate anesthesia increases seizure duration during ECT. A retrospective study. Gen Hosp Psychiatry. 1993;15:115–20.
30. Abdallah CG, Fasula M, Kelmendi B, Sanacora G, Ostroff R. Rapid antidepressant effect of ketamine in the electroconvulsive therapy setting. J ECT. 2012;28:157–61.
31. Yalcin S, Aydoğan H, Selek S, Kucuk A, Yuce HH, Karababa F, Bilgiç T. Ketofol in electroconvulsive therapy anesthesia: two stones for one bird. J Anesth. 2012;26:562–7.
32. Hoyer C, Kranaster L, Janke C, Sartorius A. Impact of the anesthetic agents ketamine, etomidate, thiopental, and propofol on seizure parameters and seizure quality in electroconvulsive therapy: a retrospective study. Eur Arch Psychiatry Clin Neurosci. 2014;264:255–61.
33. Järventausta K, Chrapek W, Kampman O, Tuohimaa K, Björkqvist M, Häkkinen H, Yli-Hankala A, Leinonen E. Effects of S-ketamine as an anesthetic adjuvant to propofol on

treatment response to electroconvulsive therapy in treatment-resistant depression: a randomized pilot study. J ECT. 2013;29:158–61.
34. Rasmussen KG, Kung S, Lapid MI, Oesterle TS, Geske JR, Nuttall GA, Oliver WC, Abenstein JP. A randomized comparison of ketamine versus methohexital anesthesia in electroconvulsive therapy. Psychiatry Res. 2014;215:362–5.
35. Yoosefi A, Sepehri AS, Kargar M, Akhondzadeh S, Sadeghi M, Rafei A, Alimadadi A, Ghaeli P. Comparing effects of ketamine and thiopental administration during electroconvulsive therapy in patients with major depressive disorder: a randomized, double-blind study. J ECT. 2014;30:15–21.
36. Boylan LS, Haskett RF, Mulsant BH, Greenberg RM, Prudic J, Spicknall K, Lisanby SH, Sackeim HA. Determinants of seizure threshold in ECT: benzodiazepine use, anesthetic dosage, and other factors. J ECT. 2000;16:3–18.
37. Bush G, Fink M, Petrides G, Dowling F, Francis A. Catatonia. II. Treatment with lorazepam and electroconvulsive therapy. Acta Psychiatr Scand. 1996;93:137–43.
38. Loimer N, Hofmann P, Chaudhry HR. Midazolam shortens seizure duration following electroconvulsive therapy. J Psychiatr Res. 1992;26:97–101.
39. Bailine SH, Safferman A, Vital-Herne J, Bernstein S. Flumazenil reversal of benzodiazepine-induced sedation for a patient with severe pre-ECT anxiety. Convuls Ther. 1994;10:65–8.
40. Strömgren LS, Dahl J, Fjeldborg N, Thomsen A. Factors influencing seizure duration and number of seizures applied in unilateral electroconvulsive therapy. Anaesthetics and benzodiazepines. Acta Psychiatr Scand. 1980;62:158–65.
41. Krystal AD, Watts BV, Weiner RD, Moore S, Steffens DC, Lindahl V. The use of flumazenil in the anxious and benzodiazepine-dependent ECT patient. J ECT. 1998;14:5–14.
42. Yi J, Torres J, Azner Y, Vaidya P, Schiavi A, Reti IM. Flumazenil pretreatment in benzodiazepine-free patients: a novel method for managing declining ECT seizure quality. J ECT. 2012;28:185–9.
43. Tanaka N, Saito Y, Hikawa Y, Nakazawa K, Yasuda K, Amaha K. Effects of thiopental and sevoflurane on hemodynamics during anesthetic management of electroconvulsive therapy. Masui. 1997;46:1575–9. Japanese.
44. Calarge CA, Crowe RR, Gergis SD, Arndt S, From RP. The comparative effects of sevoflurane and methohexital for electroconvulsive therapy. J ECT. 2003;19:221–5.
45. Toprak HI, Gedik E, Begeç Z, Oztürk E, Kaya B, Ersoy MO. Sevoflurane as an alternative anaesthetic for electroconvulsive therapy. J ECT. 2005;21:108–10.
46. Hodgson RE, Dawson P, Hold AR, Rout CC, Zuma K. Anaesthesia for electroconvulsive therapy: a comparison of sevoflurane with propofol. Anaesth Intensive Care. 2004;32:241–5.
47. Rasmussen KG, Laurila DR, Brady BM, Lewis CL, Niemeyer KD, Sun NM, Marienau ME, Hooten WM, Schroeder DR, Spackman TM. Seizure length with sevoflurane and thiopental for induction of general anesthesia in electroconvulsive therapy: a randomized double-blind trial. J ECT. 2006;22:240–2.
48. Erdil F, Begeç Z, Kayhan GE, Yoloğlu S, Ersoy MO, Durmuş M. Effects of sevoflurane or ketamine on the QTc interval during electroconvulsive therapy. J Anesth. 2014 [Epub ahead of print]
49. Lam RW. Antidepressants and QTc prolongation. J Psychiatry Neurosci. 2013;38:E5–6.
50. Dinwiddie SH, Isenberg KE. Combined alfentanil-methohexital anesthesia in electroconvulsive therapy. Convuls Ther. 1995;11:170–6.
51. Beresford BJ, Glick D, Dinwiddie SH. Combination propofol-alfentanil anesthesia for electroconvulsive therapy in patients receiving monoamine oxidase inhibitors. J ECT. 2004;20:120–2.
52. Nguyen TT, Chhibber AK, Lustik SJ, Kolano JW, Dillon PJ, Guttmacher LB. Effect of methohexitone and propofol with or without alfentanil on seizure duration and recovery in electroconvulsive therapy. Br J Anesth. 1997;79:801–3.
53. Andersen FA, Arsland D, Holst-Larsen H. Effects of combined methohexitone-remifentanil anesthesia in electroconvulsive therapy. Acta Anaesthesiol Scand. 2001;45:830–3.

54. Weinger MB, Partridge BL, Hauger R, Mirow A, Brown M. Prevention of the cardiovascular and neuroendocrine response to electroconvulsive therapy: II. Effects of pretreatment regimens on catecholamines, ACTH, vasopressin, and cortisol. Anesth Analg. 1991;73:563–9; Sackeim HA, Devanand DP, Prudic J. Stimulus intensity, seizure threshold, and seizure duration: impact on the efficacy and safety of electroconvulsive therapy. Psychiatric Clinics of North America. 1991;14:803–43.
55. Selvin BL. Electroconvulsive therapy–1987. Anesthesiology. 1987;67:367–85.
56. Stanski DR. Monitoring depth of anesthesia. In: Miller RD, editor. Anesthesia. 5th ed. Philadelphia: Churchill Livingstone; 2000. p. 1087–116.
57. Reves JG, Glass PSA, Lubarsky DA. Nonbarbiturate intravenous anesthetics. In: Miller RD, editor. Anesthesia. 5th ed. Philadelphia: Churchill Livingstone; 2000. p. 228–72.
58. Tanabe T, Sakai T, Mi WD, Matsuki A. Electroconvulsive therapy decreased bispectral index–a case report. Masui. 1998;47:1096–8.
59. Gunawardane PO, Murphy PA, Sleigh JW. Bispectral index monitoring during electroconvulsive therapy under propofol anaesthesia. Br J Anaesth. 2002;88:184–7.
60. Nishihara F, Saito S. Pre-ictal bispectral index has a positive correlation with seizure duration during electroconvulsive therapy. Anesth Analg. 2002;94:1249–52.
61. White PF, Rawal S, Recart A, Thornton L, Litle M, Stool L. Can the bispectral index be used to predict seizure time and awakening after electroconvulsive therapy? Anesth Analg. 2003;96:1636–9.
62. Lemmens HJ, Levi DC, Debattista C, Brock-Utne JG. The timing of electroconvulsive therapy and bispectral index after anesthesia induction using different drugs does not affect seizure duration. J Clin Anesth. 2003;15:29–32.
63. Fink M. Convulsive therapy: a review of the first 55 years. J Affect Disord. 2001;63:1–15.
64. Weiner RD, Coffey CD, Fochtmann LJ, et al., editors. The practice of electroconvulsive therapy; recommendations for treatment, training and privileging. 2nd ed. Washington, DC: American Psychiatric Association; 2001.
65. Nott MR, Watts JS. A fractured hip during electro-convulsive therapy. Eur J Anaesthesiol. 1999;16:265–7.
66. Sarpel Y, Toğrul E, Herdem M, Tan I, Baytok G. Central acetabular fracture-dislocation following electroconvulsive therapy: report of two similar cases. J Trauma. 1996;41:342–4.
67. Mirzakhani H, Welch CA, Eikermann M, Nozari A. Neuromuscular blocking agents for electroconvulsive therapy: a systematic review. Acta Anaesthesiol Scand. 2012;56:3–16.
68. Murali N, Saravanan ES, Ramesh VJ, Gangadhar BN, Jananakiramiah N, Kumar SS, Christopher R, Subbakrishna DK. An intrasubject comparison of two doses of succinylcholine in modified electroconvulsive therapy. Anesth Analg. 1999;89:1301–4.
69. Matsumoto N, Tomioka A, Sato T, Kawasaki M, Kadoi Y, Saito S. Relationship between cardiac output and onset of succinylcholine chloride action in electroconvulsive therapy patients. J ECT. 2009;25:246–9.
70. Williams J, Rosenquist P, Arias L, McCall WV. Pseudocholinesterase deficiency and electroconvulsive therapy. J ECT. 2007;23:198–200.
71. Cooper RC, Baumann PL, McDonald WM. An unexpected hyperkalemic response to succinylcholine during electroconvulsive therapy for catatonic schizophrenia. Anesthesiology. 1999;91:574–5.
72. Janis K, Hess J, Fabian JA, Gillis M. Substitution of mivacurium for succinylcholine for ECT in elderly patients. Can J Anaesth. 1995;42:612–3.
73. Kelly D, Brull SJ. Neuroleptic malignant syndrome and mivacurium: a safe alternative to succinylcholine? Can J Anaesth. 1994;41:845–9.
74. Cheam EW, Critchley LA, Chui PT, Yap JC, Ha VW. Low dose mivacurium is less effective than succinylcholine in electroconvulsive therapy. Can J Anaesth. 1999;46:49–51.
75. Fredman B, Smith I, d'Etienne J, White PF. Use of muscle relaxants for electroconvulsive therapy: how much is enough? Anesth Analg. 1994;78:195–6.

76. Gitlin MC, Jahr JS, Margolis MA, McCain J. Is mivacurium chloride effective in electroconvulsive therapy? A report of four cases, including a patient with myasthenia gravis. Anesth Analg. 1993;77:392–4.
77. Lui PW, Ma JY, Chan KK. Modification of tonic-clonic convulsions by atracurium in multiple-monitored electroconvulsive therapy. J Clin Anesth. 1993;5:16–21.
78. Hickey DR, O'Connor JP, Donati F. Comparison of atracurium and succinylcholine for electroconvulsive therapy in a patient with atypical plasma cholinesterase. Can J Anaesth. 1987;34:280–3.
79. Kadar AG, Kramer BA, Barth MC, White PF. Rapacuronium: an alternative to succinylcholine for electroconvulsive therapy. Anesth Analg. 2001;92:1171–2.
80. Herriot PM, Cowain T, McLeod D. Use of vecuronium to prevent suxamethonium-induced myalgia after ECT. Br J Psychiatry. 1996;168:653–4.
81. Setoyama K, Hirata T, Saeki H, Morimoto Y, Tsuruta S, Matsumoto M, Sakabe T. Anesthetic management for electroconvulsive therapy in the patients with a history of neuroleptic malignant syndrome. Masui. 2009;58:633–6. Japanese.
82. Turkkal DC, Gokmen N, Yildiz A, Iyilikci L, Gokel E, Sagduyu K, Gunerli A. A cross-over, post-electroconvulsive therapy comparison of clinical recovery from rocuronium versus succinylcholine. J Clin Anesth. 2008;20:589–93.
83. Bryson EO, Aloysi AS, Katz M, Popeo D, Kellner CH. Rocuronium as muscle relaxant for electroconvulsive therapy in a patient with adult-onset muscular dystrophy. J ECT. 2011;27: e63–4.
84. Lee C, Jahr JS, Candiotti KA, Warriner B, Zornow MH, Naguib M. Reversal of profound neuromuscular block by sugammadex administered three minutes after rocuronium: a comparison with spontaneous recovery from succinylcholine. Anesthesiology. 2009;110:1020–5.
85. Hoshi H, Kadoi Y, Kamiyama J, Nishida A, Saito H, Taguchi M, Saito S. Use of rocuronium-sugammadex, an alternative to succinylcholine, as a muscle relaxant during electroconvulsive therapy. J Anesth. 2011;25:286–90.
86. Kadoi Y, Hoshi H, Nishida A, Saito S. Comparison of recovery times from rocuronium-induced muscle relaxation after reversal with three different doses of sugammadex and succinylcholine during electroconvulsive therapy. J Anesth. 2011;25:855–9.
87. Konishi J, Suzuki T, Kondo Y, Baba M, Ogawa S. Rocuronium and sugammadex used effectively for electroconvulsive therapy in a patient with Brugada syndrome. J ECT. 2012;28:e21–2.
88. Trollor JN, Sachdev PS. Electroconvulsive treatment of neuroleptic malignant syndrome: a review and report of cases. Aust N Z J Psychiatry. 1999;33:650–9.
89. Nisijima K, Ishiguro T. Electroconvulsive therapy for the treatment of neuroleptic malignant syndrome with psychotic symptoms: a report of five cases. J ECT. 1999;15:158–63.
90. Verdura Vizcaíno EJ, Ballesteros Sanz D, Sanz-Fuentenebro J. Electroconvulsive therapy as treatment for malignant neuroleptic syndrome. Rev Psiquiatr Salud Ment. 2011;4:169–76.
91. Addonizio G, Susman VL. ECT as a treatment alternative for patients with symptoms of neuroleptic malignant syndrome. J Clin Psychiatry. 1987;48:102–5.
92. González A, Benavides J, Lema G. Anesthesia and electroconvulsive therapy: when succinylcholine is contraindicated. J ECT. 2013;29:75–6.
93. Maeda T, Enomoto T, Kamiyama Y, Inada E. Anesthetic management for electroconvulsive therapy using rocuronium bromide and sugammadex sodium in a patient with suspected malignant syndrome. Masui. 2011;60:1384–6. Japanese.

Airway and Respiratory Management During Electroconvulsive Therapy (ECT)

4

Ethan O. Bryson and Charles H. Kellner

Abstract

Electroconvulsive therapy (ECT) continues to be an important treatment modality in contemporary psychiatric medicine for severe and treatment-resistant depression and psychotic disorders. Because anesthesia technique has a particularly significant impact on the safety and efficacy of the procedure, it is critical that attention is paid to optimizing all aspects of anesthesia management. A close, collaborative working relationship between the psychiatrist and anesthesia provider is an important element in achieving optimum patient outcomes as airway and respiratory management are crucial aspects of the ECT procedure that impact both patient safety and the efficacy of the treatment. Modern ECT involves the active management of ventilation and oxygenation by an anesthesia care provider expertly trained in airway management. Pre-oxygenation followed by hyperventilation with 100 % oxygen can produce significant hypocapnia and enhance seizure activity while also increasing the period of time before significant desaturation occurs. Expert pre-procedural assessment of the patient's airway, as well as management with controlled hyperventilation during the procedure, will contribute to optimal patient outcomes.

Keywords

Anesthesia • ECT • Electroconvulsive therapy • Hyperventilation • Hyperoxia • Airway management • Respiratory management

E.O. Bryson (✉)
Departments of Anesthesiology and Psychiatry, Icahn School of Medicine at Mount Sinai, One Gustave L Levy Place, Box 1010, New York, NY 10029, USA
e-mail: ethan.bryson@mountsinai.org

C.H. Kellner
Department of Psychiatry, Division of Geriatric Psychiatry, Icahn School of Medicine at Mount Sinai, 1425 Madison Avenue 4th Floor Room 4-33, New York, NY 10029, USA
e-mail: charles.kellner@mssm.edu

S. Saito (ed.), *Anesthesia Management for Electroconvulsive Therapy*,
DOI 10.1007/978-4-431-55717-3_4

4.1 Introduction

Electroconvulsive therapy (ECT) continues to be an important treatment modality in contemporary psychiatric medicine for severe and treatment-resistant depression and psychotic disorders. Because anesthesia technique has a particularly significant impact on the safety and efficacy of the procedure, it is critical that attention is paid to optimizing all aspects of anesthesia management. A close, collaborative working relationship between the psychiatrist and anesthesia provider is an important element in achieving optimum patient outcomes.

Modern ECT involves the active management of ventilation and oxygenation by an anesthesia care provider expertly trained in airway management. Pre-oxygenation followed by hyperventilation with 100 % oxygen can produce significant hypocapnia and enhance seizure activity while also increasing the period of time before significant desaturation occurs. For the vast majority of patients, the airway can be properly managed with a manual self-inflating bag-valve-mask device (Fig. 4.1). Some patients may require an oral airway (Fig. 4.2), and in rare instances some may require the use of a laryngeal mask airway (LMA) (Fig. 4.3) or endotracheal tube (ETT) (Fig. 4.4). Though it is the rare patient who requires intubation, since general anesthesia is administered as part of ECT, the physician anesthesiologist or certified registered nurse anesthetist (CRNA) should always be prepared to secure the airway with an endotracheal tube, either electively prior to the treatment or emergently after the induction of anesthesia if ventilation is not possible by other means.

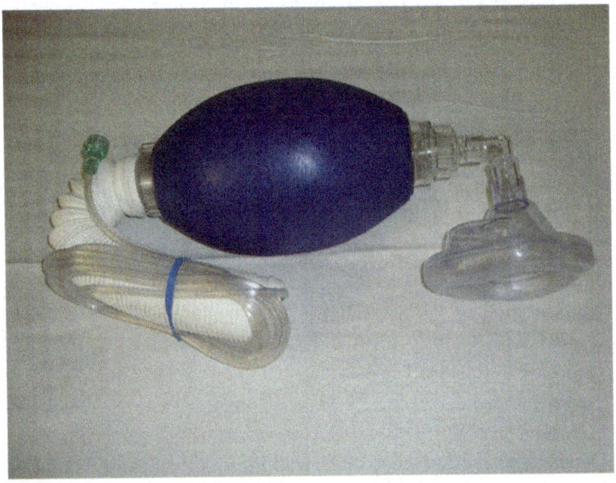

Fig. 4.1 Manual self-inflating bag-valve-mask device, removed from packaging. Note that for this model the accordion reservoir must be extended prior to use

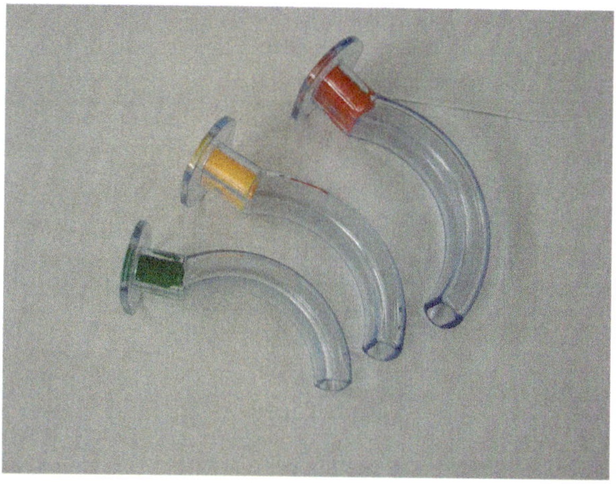

Fig. 4.2 Various size oral airways

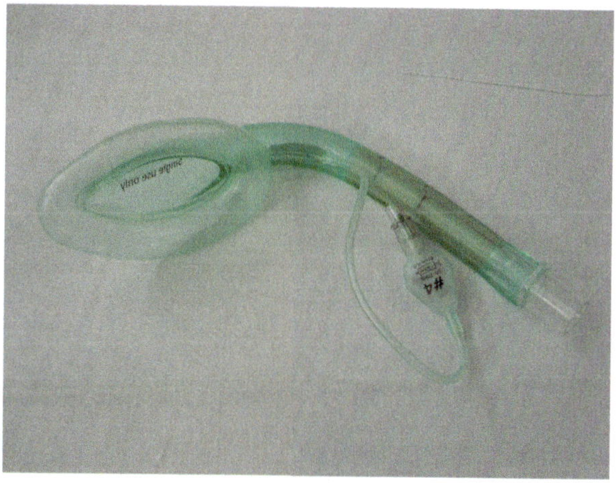

Fig. 4.3 laryngeal mask airway

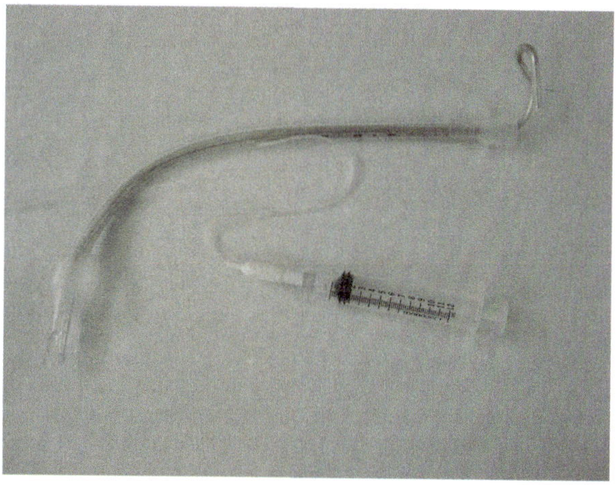

Fig. 4.4 Endotracheal tube with intubating stylette inserted and cuff inflated

4.2 Airway Management

The ability to manage a patient's airway is dependent upon proper assessment prior to the initiation of therapy. Identification of the patient with a potentially difficult airway, that is, one who might be difficult to ventilate or intubate, can avoid significant morbidity or mortality. It should be noted here that factors which make a patient potentially difficult to ventilate or intubate may overlap but are not all the same, and the misidentification of these factors can have significant consequences.

4.2.1 Assessment

Evaluation of the patients' airway begins with the patient in the sitting position facing forward, toward the evaluator (Fig. 4.5). Note the patient's neck size and presence or absence of redundant soft tissue externally, which may indicate internal redundant soft tissue, or facial hair, both of which may make mask ventilation difficult [1]. Ask the patient to open their mouth as wide as they can and measure the distance between the mandibular and maxillary incisors. An inter-incisor distance of less than 6 cm has been associated with a difficult-to-intubate patient [2]. If the patient cannot open their mouth more than 3 cm and requires placement of an oral airway, ventilation may be difficult as well [3]. If the patient is edentulous, it may be difficult to form an air-tight seal with a mask. Ask the patient to extend their tongue as far as possible (Fig. 4.6). It is important that they do not phonate for this part of the exam. Often patients will spontaneously say "Ahh" as

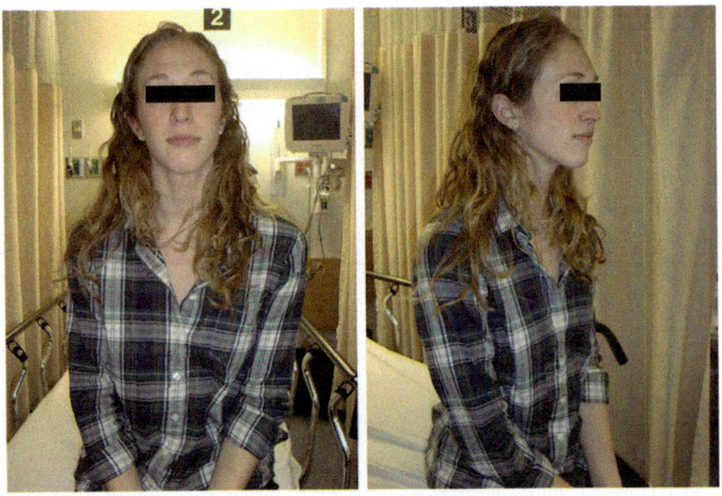

Fig. 4.5 Proper position for airway evaluation. The patient should be sitting upright, facing forward. Note that many patients are assessed while lying down on a stretcher and in this situation should be asked to sit upright, preferably at the edge of the stretcher

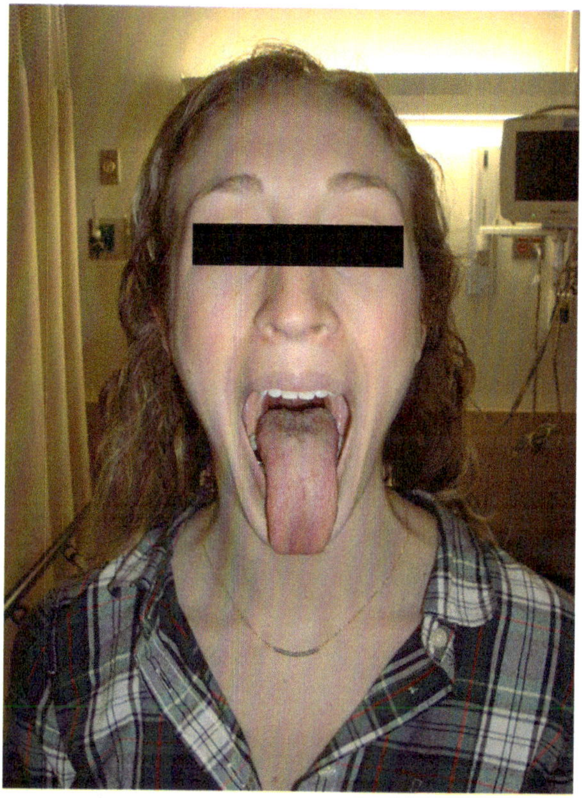

Fig. 4.6 Once the patient is positioned properly, ask them to open their mouth as wide as possible and extrude their tongue. Many patients will spontaneously phonate at this point, ask that they do not say "Ahh" as this will lift the soft palate, and erroneously decrease the Mallampati score

this is what most doctors have asked them to do when they have been instructed to open their mouths in the past, but phonating will lift the soft palate and may generate a falsely low Mallampati classification score (Fig. 4.7). The Mallampati score is used to evaluate the potential for a difficult intubation [4]. Higher Mallampati scores are predictive of difficulty with intubation and are also associated with an increased risk of sleep apnea and difficult ventilation [5]. Generating a Mallampati score involves identifying the internal structures of the oropharynx and their relation to each other. Specifically, look to see whether the base of the uvula, faucial pillars (the arches in front of and behind the tonsils), and soft palate are visible.

The modified Mallampati scoring system as described by Samsoon and Young [6] is the most widely used classification system:

- Class I: Soft palate, uvula, fauces, pillars visible.
- Class II: Soft palate, uvula, fauces visible.
- Class III: Soft palate, base of uvula visible.
- Class IV: Only hard palate visible

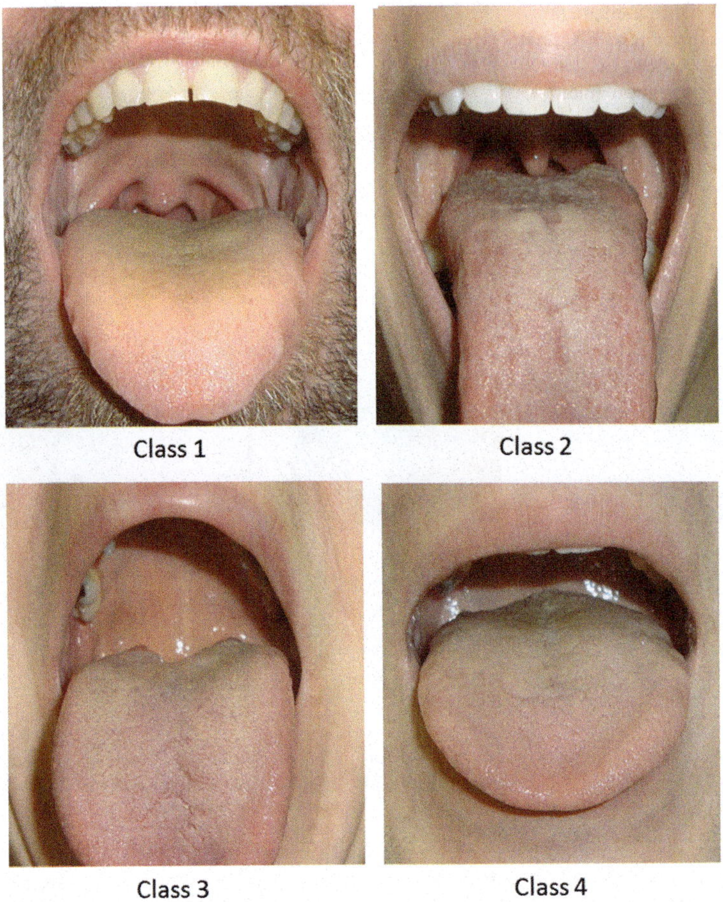

Fig. 4.7 Mallampati score chart. In the class 1 airway the soft palate, uvula, fauces, and pillars are visible. In the class 2 airway the soft palate, uvula and fauces are visible but the tonsillar pillars are not. In the class 3 airway, only the soft palate and the base of uvula are visible. In the class 4 airway, only the hard palate is visible

Now turn your attention to the jaw and examine the mandible from the side (Fig. 4.8). Measure the thyro-mental distance, which is the distance between the thyroid cartilage and the tip of the mandible. This distance should be at least 6.5 cm. Shorter thyro-mental distances are associated with a potentially difficult intubation as there is less room to displace the base of the tongue and associated soft tissue structures during direct laryngoscopy.

By themselves, none of these factors can always predict that a patient will be difficult to ventilate or to intubate; rather, taken together, they are used to generate a clinical picture of the patient, which the expert in airway management can use to choose the safest way to anesthetize the patient for the procedure. Factors that are

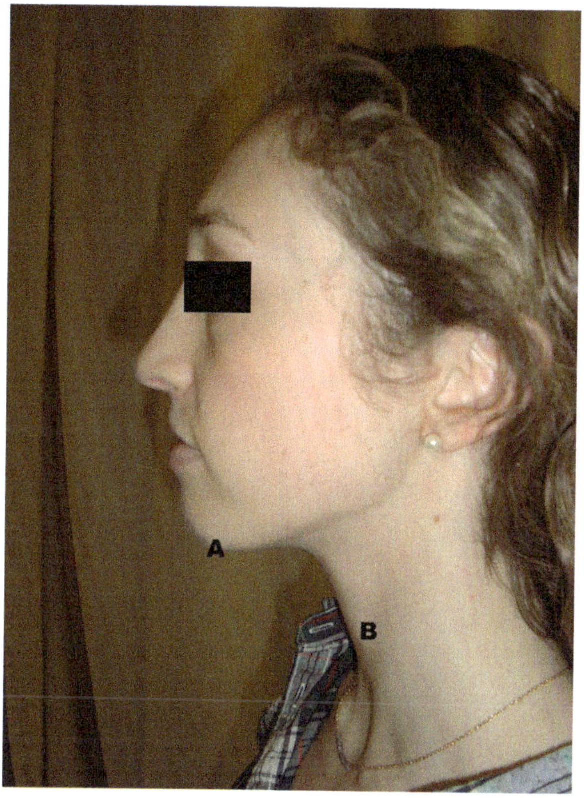

Fig. 4.8 The thyro-mental distance is the distance between the thyroid cartilage (**b**) and the tip of the mandible (**a**). This distance should be at least 6.5 cm

associated with difficult ventilation and/or difficult intubation are listed in Table 4.1 for comparison.

4.2.2 Management Techniques

As stated earlier, the vast majority of patients' airways can be effectively managed using only a manual self-inflating bag-valve-mask device. The mask should be held in place over the patient's nose and mouth with the thumb and first finger while the patient's face is lifted into the mask by placing the remaining fingers along the mandible and applying a pulling pressure. Care should be taken to minimize the motion of the cervical spine, especially in patients with arthritis or cervical spine disease. Simply pressing the mask down onto the patient's face can cause the base of the tongue to obstruct the airway and result in the need for higher pressures during positive pressure ventilation. It is important to qualitatively judge the insufflation pressures required to effectively ventilate during the first or second breath, as pressures above 19 cm H_2O can overcome the static pressure of the lower esophageal sphincter muscle, leading to insufflation of the stomach. Over inflation

Table 4.1 Factors associated with difficult ventilation versus difficult intubation:

Predictor	Difficult ventilation	Difficult intubation
Mouth opening < 3 cm	X	X
Limited neck movement		X
Mallampati score III–IV		X
Thyromental distance < 6 cm		X
Neck circumference > 43 cm	X	X
Presence of beard	X	
Edentulous	X	
Obstructive sleep apnea	X	X

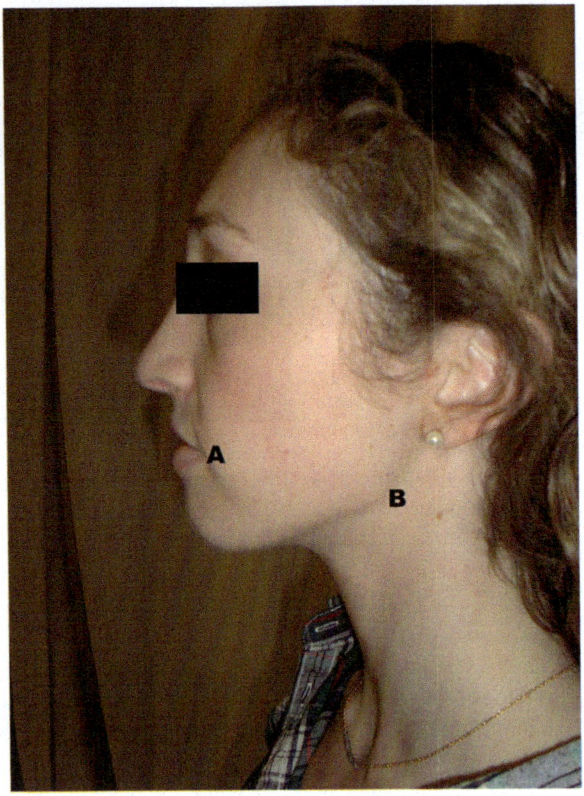

Fig. 4.9 The appropriate size oral airway can quickly be estimated by using the device to measure the distance from the corner of the mouth (**a**) to the angle of the mandible (**b**)

can lead to reflexive emptying of gastric contents and subsequent aspiration and should be avoided. If difficulty with ventilation is encountered, immediate placement of an oral airway is indicated. It is important to choose the appropriate size oral airway. This can quickly be estimated by using the airway to measure the distance from the corner of the mouth to the angle of the mandible (Fig. 4.9). Often this will relieve the obstruction and allow for proper ventilation. In rare instances, when the patient cannot be ventilated with a properly sized oral airway in place, an

LMA must be placed or the patient must be intubated. In these instances, care must be taken to place a modified bite-block around the LMA or ETT prior to stimulus application.

4.2.3 Who Needs to Be Intubated for ECT?

It is the rare patient who requires endotracheal intubation for ECT anesthesia, but there are some circumstances under which this becomes necessary. Those patients who require intubation for ECT are either at significant risk of aspiration, that is, they are considered to have a "full stomach" despite having had nothing by mouth (NPO) for the recommended 8 h for solids and 2 h for clear liquids, or considered to be at significant risk for difficult ventilation and "loss of the airway" after induction of anesthesia. Patients at significantly increased risk of pulmonary aspiration despite strict adherence to NPO guidelines include patients with a bowel obstruction, motility disorders, abnormal esophageal, and gastric or bowel anatomy and patients who are actively vomiting. In each of these cases, however, it is probably more appropriate to delay ECT until these medical problems have been addressed. Patients at significant risk of difficult ventilation include the morbidly obese with a central distribution of adipose tissue, patients with a history of difficult ventilation, and pregnant patients beyond 20 weeks' gestation.

4.3 Ventilation Management

The effectiveness of ECT is intimately dependent upon the management of the patient by the anesthesiologist assisting with the procedure. Because most anesthetic agents are anticonvulsant and may raise the seizure threshold, the choice of induction agent and the actual dose administered have the potential to either enhance or degrade the quality of the seizure. Proper airway management with hyperventilation has the potential to significantly alter the treatment course of any given patient undergoing ECT by decreasing the necessity for increasing the electric charge because of inadequate seizure length [7], reducing the need for re-stimulation because of abortive seizures [8], and reducing the potential for post-ictal delirium. This technique, however, also has the potential for generating prolonged seizures in susceptible patients [9].

4.3.1 Hypocapnia

Hypocapnia achieved through hyperventilation has long been used to enhance seizure quality, is used as an activation method in standard electroencephalography for the provocation of epileptic activity [10], and is most important in patients with a higher seizure threshold or a history of inadequate seizure length [11]. Typical ETCO2 levels achieved during the period of hyperventilation prior to ECT stimulation via BVM device at a rate of 40–45 breaths per minute are commonly well below the 30 mmHg levels associated with adequate seizure enhancement. This effect of seizure enhancement is thought to be a result of the hypocapnia and subsequent respiratory alkalosis generated through hyperventilation, and not due to changes related to varying oxygen (O_2) tension [12]. Recent investigations into this method have focused on controlled hyperventilation (CHV) and its effect on multiple parameters associated with seizure efficacy and involve quantitative measurements of $ETCO_2$ during treatment [13]. In the majority of cases, hyperventilation during ECT is performed using a BVM device without a reliable seal. In this situation, while the presence or absence of $ETCO_2$ can be detected, an accurate value cannot be detected. In these studies, however, the goal was to reduce the CO_2 level to below a partial pressure of 30 millimeters of mercury (mmHg), and the patients were ventilated using a device which specifically isolated the patients' lungs from the atmosphere, thus providing an accurate measurement of $ETCO_2$. This technique has been shown to improve seizure parameters typically associated with antidepressant efficacy, leading to a decreased need to increase stimulus intensity, a decreased need to re-stimulate, and fewer treatments needed to induce remission.

Though many studies support the use of hyperventilation, the level of contribution to seizure parameter improvement has been questioned by some investigators [14]. Several confounding variables, other than $ETCO_2$, with the potential to independently alter seizure parameters have been identified in these investigations. The choice of anesthetic and anesthetic dose are obvious ones, but even the period of time between the end of hyperventilation and the application of the stimulus has been implicated as a variable with the potential to change seizure efficacy.

Given the considerable data which suggests that controlled hyperventilation in patients receiving ECT can lead to more effective treatment, it is important to examine the physiological consequences of reduced CO_2 levels. Hyperventilation is known to increase cerebrovascular resistance (CVR), leading to a reduction in cerebral blood flow (CBF), decreased cerebral oxygen delivery (cDO_2), and impaired cerebral metabolism to a degree depending on the level of $ETCO_2$ achieved [15]. Under the conditions of mild hyperventilation ($ETCO_2$ reduced to 30 mmHg), CBF is reduced by 60 % and cDO_2 by 58 % in patients with normal cerebral physiology [16]. While at this level cerebral metabolic rate for oxygen and glucose is not altered, the net cerebral lactate efflux is increased, suggesting a partial impairment of cerebral aerobic metabolism. Patients with altered cerebral physiology, such as patients with Alzheimer's disease, neurotrauma, meningitis, and other vascular disorders, are known to have an increased vasoconstrictive response to hypocapnia, which could potentially magnify this effect [17, 18, 19, 20, 21, 22]. Some investigators have suggested that the common practice of inducing intraoperative hyperventilation (in procedures other than ECT) may be deleterious and result in increased length of stay for post-operative patients, though the clinical implications of a short period of hypoventilation during ECT are unclear [23].

4.3.2 Hyperoxia

Current standard ECT practice prior to induction of general anesthesia includes pre-oxygenation via either nasal cannula oxygen or face mask, depending on what can be tolerated by the individual patient [24]. These devices must be removed prior to providing positive pressure ventilation via BVM device, but this is generally a simple procedure with little downside, provided the ECT recording electrodes are not disturbed in the process. This practice not only improves the safety of the procedure by increasing the oxygen reserves of the patient and thus increasing the period of tolerable apnea, but hyperoxia may also improve seizure quality [25]. Passive pre-oxygenation with either a nasal cannula or a face mask is followed by active hyperventilation with 100 % oxygen via BVM device, further increasing the blood oxygen partial pressures.

Hyperoxia in certain situations, such as artificially created undersea environments, may be toxic and induce spontaneous seizures when it is present in partial pressures above atmospheric norms [26]. Specific benefits of hyperoxia in ECT include the potential to reduce the stimulus charge needed to elicit an adequate seizure, as well as seizure prolongation and enhanced EEG expression of the seizure [27].

4.3.3 Conclusion

Airway and respiratory management are crucial aspects of the ECT procedure that impact both patient safety and the efficacy of the treatment. Expert pre-procedural assessment of the patient's airway, as well as management with controlled hyperventilation during the procedure, will contribute to optimal patient outcomes.

References

1. Kheterpal S, Healy D, Aziz MF, Shanks AM, Freundlich RE, Linton F, Martin LD, Linton J, Epps JL, Fernandez-Bustamante A, Jameson LC, Tremper T, Tremper KK, Multicenter Perioperative Outcomes Group (MPOG) Perioperative Clinical Research Committee. Incidence, predictors, and outcome of difficult mask ventilation combined with difficult laryngoscopy: a report from the multicenter perioperative outcomes group. Anesthesiology. 2013;119(6):1360–9.
2. Wilson ME, Spiegelhalter D, Robertson JA, Lesser P. Predicting difficult intubation. Br J Anesth. 1988;61:211–6.
3. Shah PJ, Dubey KP, Yadav JP. Predictive value of upper lip bite test and ratio of height to thyromental distance compared to other multivariate airway assessment tests for difficult laryngoscopy in apparently normal patients. J Anaesthesiol Clin Pharmacol. 2013;29:191–5.
4. Mallampati SR, Gatt SP, Gugino LD, Desai SP, Waraksa B, Freiberger D, Liu PL. A clinical sign to predict difficult tracheal intubation: a prospective study. Can Anaesth Soc J. 1985;32(4):429–34.
5. Nuckton TJ, Glidden DV, Browner WS, Claman DM. Physical examination: Mallampati score as an independent predictor of obstructive sleep apnea. Sleep. 2006;29(7):903–8.

6. Samsoon GL, Young JR. Difficult tracheal intubation: a retrospective study. Anaesthesia. 1987;42(5):487–90.
7. Bergshlom P, Gran L, Bleie H. Seizure duration in unilateral electroconvulsive therapy. The effect of Hypocapnia induced hyperventilation and the effect of ventilation with oxygen. Acta Psychiatr Scand. 1984;69(2):121–8.
8. Datto C, Rai AK, Ilivicky HJ, Caroff SN. Augmentation of seizure induction in electroconvulsive therapy: a clinical reappraisal. J ECT. 2002;18(13):117.
9. Pande AC, Shea J, Shettar S. Effect of hyperventilation on seizure length during electroconvulsive therapy. Biol Psychiatry. 1990;27(7):799–801.
10. Weiner RD. The psychiatric use of electrically induced seizures. Am J Psychiatry. 1979;136:1507–17.
11. Chater SN, Simpson KH. Effect of passive hyperventilation on seizure duration in patients undergoing electroconvulsive therapy. Br J Anaesth. 1988;60(1):70–3.
12. Bergsholm P, Gran L, Bleie H. Seizure duration in unilateral electroconvulsive therapy. The effect of hypocapnia induced by hyperventilation and the effect of ventilation with oxygen. Acta Psychiatr Scand. 1984;69(2):121–8.
13. Haeck M, Gillmann B, Janouscheck H, Grozinger M. Electroconvulsive therapy can benefit from controlled hyperventilation using a laryngeal mask. Eur Arch Psychiatry Clin Neurosci. 2011;261 Suppl 2:S172–6.
14. Sawayama E, Takhashi M, Inoue A. Moderate hyperventilation prolongs electroencephalogram seizure duration of the first electroconvulsive therapy. J ECT. 2008;24(3):195–8.
15. Brian Jr JE. Carbon dioxide and the cerebral circulation. Anesthesiology. 1998;88:1356–86.
16. Grune F, Kazmaier S, Sonntag H, Stolker RJ, Weyland A. Moderate hyperventilation during intravenous anesthesia increases net cerebral lactate efflux. Anesthesiology. 2014;120:335–42.
17. Nagata K, Buchan RJ, Yokoyama E, Kondoh Y, Sato M, Terashi H, Satoh Y, Watahiki Y, Senova M, Hirata Y, Hatazawa J. Misery perfusion with preserved vascular reactivity in Alzheimer's disease. Ann NY Acad Sci. 1997;826:272–81.
18. Meyer JS, Sawada T, Kitamura A, Toyoda M. Cerebral oxygen, glucose, lactate, and pyruvate metabolism in stroke, therapeutic considerations. Circulation. 1968;37:1036–48.
19. Robertson CS, Narayan RK, Gokaslan ZI, Pahwa R, Grossman RG, Caram Jr P, Allen E. Cerebral arteriovenous oxygen difference as an estimate of cerebral blood flow in comatose patients. J Neurosurg. 1989;70:222–30.
20. Thees C, Scholz M, Schaller MDC, Gass A, Pavlidis C, Weyland A, Hoeft A. Relationship between intracranial pressure and critical closing pressure in patients with neurotrauma. Anesthesiology. 2002;96:595–9.
21. Coles JP, Minhas PS, Fryer TD, Smielewski P, Aigbirihio F, Donovan T, Downey SP, Williams G, Chatfield D, Matthwes JC, Gupta AK, Carpenter TA, Clark JC, Pickard JD, Menon DK. Effect of hyperventilation on cerebral blood flow in traumatic head injury: clinical relevance and monitoring correlates. Crit Care Med. 2002;30:1950–9.
22. Moller K, Strauss GI, Thomsen G, Larsen FS, Holm S, Sperling BK, Skinhoj P, Knudsen GM. Cerebral blood flow, oxidative metabolism and cerebrovascular Carbon dioxide reactivity in patients with acute bacterial meningitis. Acta Anesthesiol Scand. 2002;46:567–78.
23. Wax DB, Lin HM, Hossain S, Porter SB. Intraoperative carbon dioxide management and outcomes. Eur J Anesthesiol. 2010;27:819–23.
24. Kellner CH, Bryson EO. Electroconvulsive therapy anesthesia technique: minimalist versus maximally managed. J ECT. 2013;29:153–5.
25. Aksay SS, Bumb JM, Janke C, Hoyer C, Kranaster L, Sartorious A. New evidence for seizure quality improvement by hyperoxia and mild hypocapnia. JECT. 2015;30(4):287–91.
26. Wood JD. Oxygen toxicity. In: Bennet PB, Elliot EH, editors. Physiology and medicine of diving and compressed air work. London: Balliere Tindall & Cassell; 1975. p. 166–84.
27. Loo CK, Mahon M, Katalinic N. Predictors of response to ultrabrief right unilateral electroconvulsive therapy. J Affec Disord. 2011;130:192–7.

Circulatory Management, Especially Blood Pressure and Heart Rate

5

Naoki Matsumoto

Abstract

Recent guidelines have stated that anesthesia for electroconvulsive therapy (ECT) should be administered by a specially trained anesthesiologist, and that anesthesiologists have overall responsibility, not only for anesthesia itself, but also for cardiopulmonary management and emergency care. Accordingly, anesthesiologists who administer anesthesia for ECT should have sufficient knowledge regarding the unique physiological and pharmacological effects of ECT. The electrical current during ECT stimulates the autonomic nervous system and provokes unique hemodynamic changes in systemic and cerebral circulation. Excessive alterations in heart rate, blood pressure, and cardiac function should be prevented by drugs, such as anticholinergic and antihypertensive agents. Ventilation should be adequately maintained to ensure the efficacy of the therapy and to stabilize hemodynamics immediately after the electrical stimulation. Reports of serious complications of this therapy are not frequent; however, patients with ischemic heart disease or cerebrovascular problems must be managed with special care to prevent myocardial infarction or neurological disorders. Safe physical management by anesthesiologists greatly contributes to the safety of ECT under muscle relaxation. To maintain social confidence and to refine the therapy, anesthesiologists should play an essential role in both clinical application and laboratory research on ECT.

Keywords

Circulatory management • Blood pressure • Heart rate • Beta-blocker • Ca^{2+}-channel antagonists

N. Matsumoto (✉)
Department of Anesthesia, Gunma Children's Medical Center, 779 Shimohakoda, Hokkitsu, Shibukawa, Gunma 377-8577, Japan
e-mail: nmatsumoto@gunma-u.ac.jp

S. Saito (ed.), *Anesthesia Management for Electroconvulsive Therapy*,
DOI 10.1007/978-4-431-55717-3_5

5.1 Introduction

Electroconvulsive therapy (ECT) was introduced in clinical practice based on the observation that psychiatric symptoms in patients with both schizophrenia and epilepsy were improved after a seizure. However, in spite of the great effort expended, the underlying mechanism for this has not been fully elucidated [1, 2]. ECT therapy has undergone several decades of criticism, accusations of inappropriate use, legal restrictions, and public protest [3]. However, recent controlled studies have demonstrated the clinical benefits of this therapy, and many efforts have been made to reduce the special risks of ECT [4, 5]. Specifically, the introduction of general anesthesia using intravenous anesthetics and a muscle relaxant has greatly reduced the physical risks related to the convulsive muscular movements during the therapy. Currently, ECT for drug therapy-resistant depression and some other psychiatric disorders is widely accepted as safe and effective therapy.

However, ECT may be associated with significant cardiovascular morbidity and mortality [6–8]. For example, 35 cardiac arrests during ECT were reported in California from 1974 to 1983 [7], and the cardiovascular mortality of this procedure has been reported to be as high as 0.03 % [8]. The cardiac morbidity of ECT is usually due to arrhythmias and lability of arterial blood pressure, resulting in myocardial infarction, congestive heart failure, cardiac arrest, and/or cerebrovascular events.

Although the basic mechanism of the clinical effects of ECT has not been clarified, several authorized medical societies, including the Royal College of Psychiatrists in the United Kingdom [9] and the American Psychiatric Association [10], have published guidelines and audit reports to promote the safe and effective use of ECT and to prevent its misuse. The most recent version of the guideline by the American Psychiatric Association clearly states that anesthesia for ECT should be administered by a specially trained anesthesiologist and that the anesthesiologists have overall responsibility, not only for anesthesia itself, but also for cardiopulmonary management and emergency care [10, 11]. Accordingly, anesthesiologists who administer anesthesia for ECT should have sufficient knowledge regarding the unique physiological and pharmacological effects of ECT.

5.2 Hemodynamic Variations

5.2.1 Mechanism

The electrical current during ECT stimulates the autonomic nervous system and provokes unique hemodynamic changes in the systemic circulation [12, 13]. First, a parasympathetic upsurge occurs immediately after the application of electrical current; this phase ensues within a few seconds. Second, sympathetic systems are stimulated and catecholamines are released from the adrenal medulla and sympathetic nerve terminals [14]. This phase continues for approximately 10 min. Several

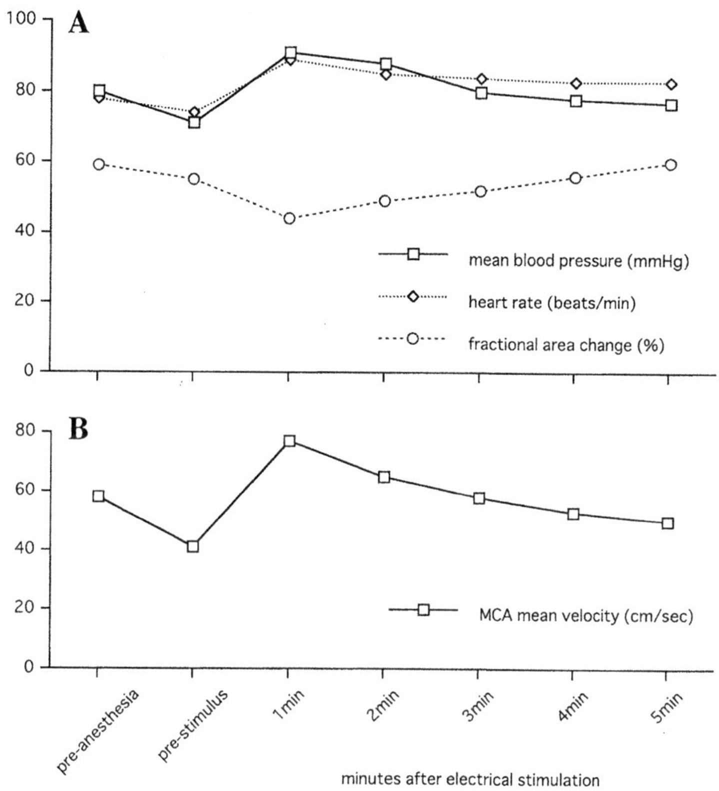

Fig. 5.1 Typical changes in systemic and cerebral hemodynamics in a patient. (**a**) Typical changes in heart rate, blood pressure, and fractional area change. (**b**) Typical change in cerebral blood flow velocity measured in the middle cerebral artery (MCA) (From Saito et al. [15]. Used with permission)

unique hemodynamic changes are provoked by the sequential autonomic activation (Fig. 5.1) [15].

Selection of anesthetics and determination of the dose of the selected anesthetic are crucial in ECT management, because these factors have a potent impact on heart rate, blood pressure, cerebral blood flow, and seizure induction in ECT (Table 5.1).

5.2.2 Heart Rate

Patients presenting for ECT may have tachycardia before the therapy due to dehydration induced by difficulty in oral intake [10, 16]. Vasodilatory intravenous anesthetics, such as thiopental, provoke a further increase in heart rate [17]. In contrast, propofol maintains a stable heart rate or decreases the heart rate to some extent [17]. Parasympathetic discharge immediately after electrical stimulation suppresses the heart rate [18]. In some patients, the bradycardia is severe, and

Table 5.1 Effects of anesthetics when used during ECT

	Heart rate	Blood pressure	Cerebral blood flow	Seizure duration	Others
Methohexital	→/↑	↓/↑↑	N.E.	→	Standard anesthetic for ECT
Thiopental	↑/↑	↓/↑↑	↓/↑↑	↓	Histamine release
Propofol	↓/↑→	↓/↑	↓/↑	↓	Injection pain
Diazepam	→/↑	↓/↑	N.E.	↓↓	Long acting
Ketamine	↑/↑	↑/↑↑	↑/↑↑	↑↓	Psychotic action
Etomidate	→/↑	→/↑↑	N.E.	↑	Injection pain, slow recovery
Sevoflurane	↑/↑	↓/↑	↑/↑↑	↓↓	Slow induction

From Saito et al. [15]. Used with permission
Effects of anesthetics before and after electrical stimulation (before electrical stimulation/after electrical stimulation)

temporary asystole might be observed [19–21]. However, this phase passes within a minute and the subsequent sympathetic activation induces tachycardia. If a patient has an arrhythmogenic tendency, dysrhythmia might be provoked in this phase [22]. This tachycardia is augmented by excessive hypocarbia induced by deliberate hyperventilation [23], hypercarbia induced by inappropriate ventilation [24], use of vasodilatory antihypertensive drugs [17], or prolonged seizure activity [25]. In appropriately managed patients, this tachycardia phase lasts for 2–5 min [24].

5.2.3 Blood Pressure

Many patients who use psychotropic drugs are relatively hypotensive [26]. If the patient also has a problem with food intake, the hypotension can be aggravated by dehydration. Intravenous anesthetics used in ECT, except for ketamine and etomidate, induce temporary hypotension due to their vasodilatory and myocardial depressant properties [17]. However, sympathetic stimulation by the electrical current and the subsequent catecholamine increase overshadow the hypotensive effects and elevate blood pressure by 20–50 % as compared to prestimulus values [12, 27]. The elevated blood pressure gradually decreases within 2–5 min when the patient is appropriately ventilated [24]. If hypercapnea and/or hypoxia exist because of inappropriate respiratory management, the initial sympathetic stimulation may not ensue, or the elevated blood pressure persists until full recovery of spontaneous breathing [24].

5.2.4 Cardiac Function

Although the parasympathetic dominant phase immediately after electrical stimulation suppresses cardiac function, this phase lasts for only a minute, which limits the associated cardiac risk [10]. Only when the parasympathetic discharge is not counteracted by a sympathetic surge due to subconvulsive stimulation does severe bradycardia or asystole persist. In contrast, tachycardia and hypertension provoked by the subsequent sympathetic stimulation profoundly increase myocardial oxygen demand for several minutes and possibly induce myocardial ischemia in patients with compromised coronary circulation [28]. Rate pressure product, which is the product of heart rate and systolic blood pressure and is considered an indicator of myocardial oxygen demand, is increased by 50–400 % during the sympathetic dominant phase [23, 29]. Electrocardiographic ischemia is also observed in some cases [30, 31]. One echocardiographic study [30] demonstrated regional wall motion abnormalities immediately after ECT. Further, systolic performance, as indicated by fractional area change, is suppressed by tachycardia, increased systemic vascular resistance, and hypertension [32, 33] (Table 5.2).

5.2.5 Reported Complications

Since ECT provokes drastic changes in hemodynamic variables, as noted above, several fatal complications have been reported in previous literature. Cardiac arrest, probably induced by parasympathetic hyperactivity and use of a beta-blocking agent, was reported by Decina et al. [19]. Myocardial infarction and cardiac rupture were independently reported by Lopez-Gomez et al. [34] and Ali and Tidmarsh, respectively [35]. Although the incidence of such severe complications is rare [36], anesthesiologists who bear responsibility for hemodynamic management during ECT should pay special attention to the patients' cardiac risk factors of ECT during the preanesthesia physical assessment. Also, patients and/or their responsible relatives should be notified of the unique hemodynamic effects and risks of ECT.

5.2.6 Cerebral Circulation

Electrical stimulation of the brain provokes unique alterations in cerebrovascular dynamics. In the 1970s, Brodersen et al. [37] first reported cerebral hyperemia following electrically induced seizures using xenon-133. In the 1990s, Saito et al. [38, 39] and Vollmer-Hasse et al. [40] continuously measured intracranial blood flow during ECT, using real-time monitoring systems, such as transcranial Doppler ultrasonography and near-infrared spectrophotometry. In these studies, it was demonstrated that cerebral blood flow decreased for a few seconds immediately after electrical stimulation and then drastically increased for a few minutes (Fig. 5.1b). Since these responses are observed even after abortive stimulation, the electrical current itself (rather than seizure activity) may provoke the responses [38]. This augmented cerebral blood flow is possibly induced by the increased oxygen demand of brain tissues and the increased cerebral perfusion pressure secondary to systemic hyperdynamic responses [39]. The degree of cerebral hyperemia has a positive correlation with the degree of systemic blood pressure elevation

Table 5.2 Time course of changes in hemodynamic variables

Measurement time	(1)	(2)	(3)	(4)	(5)	(6)	(7)	(8)
End-diastolic area (cm^2)	7.5 ± 0.8	7.8 ± 0.8	9.3 ± 0.9	8.2 ± 0.7	8.4 ± 0.9	8.8 ± 0.6	8.9 ± 0.8	7.8 ± 0.7
End-systolic area (cm^2)	3.1 ± 0.3	3.5 ± 0.4	5.5 ± 0.6*	4.7 ± 0.4	4.1 ± 0.6	4.0 ± 0.4	3.7 ± 0.4	3.4 ± 0.4
Fractional area change (%)	58 ± 5	55 ± 4	44 ± 4*	49 ± 5	52 ± 5	56 ± 4	60 ± 5	56 ± 4
Heart rate (beat · min^{-1})	92 ± 5	91 ± 6	106 ± 7	104 ± 7	99 ± 5	97 ± 4	96 ± 5	97 ± 4
Systolic BP (mmHg)	112 ± 4	108 ± 4	147 ± 10*	145 ± 6*	144 ± 7*	137 ± 6*	131 ± 6	121 ± 4
Diastolic BP (mmHg)	61 ± 4	63 ± 3	81 ± 8*	87 ± 8*	80 ± 8*	80 ± 5	73 ± 4	65 ± 3
Systolic BP/EDA-ESA	47 ± 17	48 ± 10	62 ± 11	57 ± 9	57 ± 11	55 ± 17	49 ± 13	48 ± 12

Values are expressed as mean ± SEM

EDA end-diastolic area, *ESA* end-systolic area, *HR* heart rate, *BP* blood pressure

(1) awake; (2) 1 min after propofol administration; (3) 1 min after electrical shock; (4) 2 min after electrical shock; (5) 3 min after electrical shock; (6) 4 min after electrical shock; (7) 5 min after electrical shock; (8) 10 min after electrical shock

*$P < 0.05$ compared to period (1) (From Kadoi et al. [32]. Used with permission)

Table 5.3 Effects of hemodynamic modulators when used during electroconvulsive therapy (ECT)

	Cerebral blood flow	Seizure duration
Nicardipine	↑[a]	→
Verapamil	N.E.	→
Diltiazem	N.E.	↓
Trinitroglycerine	↑→	→
Alprenolol	↑→	→
Prostaglandin E1	↑[a]	→
Labetalol	N.E.	↓→
Landiolol	↑[a]	→
Esmolol	↑[a]	↓→

From Saito et al. [15]. Used with permission
N.E. not evaluated
[a]Elevation as non-medication

[39]. Recently, Fabbri et al. [41] demonstrated that this phenomenon is not only observed with bilateral ECT, but also with unilateral ECT.

Since cerebrovascular hemodynamic alteration during ECT is partly provoked by systemic hemodynamic changes, antihypertensive regimens that prevent systemic hypertension during ECT ameliorate the cerebrovascular hemodynamic alterations to some extent [42]. However, although antihypertensive medication can prevent systemic hypertension, it cannot completely suppress reactive acceleration in middle cerebral artery blood flow. Relative effects on systemic and cerebral circulation are not identical among antihypertensive drugs (see Table 5.3). For example, the beta-blocking agent, alprenolol, and glyceryl trinitrate suppress both systemic and cerebral hemodynamics; in contrast, the calcium channel blocker, nicardipine, and prostaglandin E1 suppress mainly systemic hemodynamics and have minimal effects on cerebral hemodynamics. The choice of anesthetic agent also influences cerebrovascular reaction during ECT. The increase in middle cerebral artery blood flow velocity is minor under propofol compared to thiopental anesthesia [43]. Several authors [44–46] have speculated that the reactive hyperemia may help compensate for the increased oxygen and energy demand after electrical stimulation. Therefore, complete suppression of cerebral hyperemia may be unnecessary or inadequate for hemodynamic management during ECT.

5.2.7 Cerebrovascular Complications

Considering the abrupt changes in cerebral circulation after electrical stimulation, the presence of cerebral aneurysms and intracranial mass lesions are listed as relative contraindications of ECT in some articles [12, 47, 48]. However, case reports describing unsuccessful management of ECT in patients with cerebral complications are limited [49]. In contrast, safe completion of the therapy schedule with deliberate hemodynamic management has been reported [50–56]. Even though there are few previously reported catastrophic cases, anesthesiologists should take special care to stabilize hemodynamics and cautiously inspect neurological symptoms when ECT is administered for such patients.

5.3 Circulatory Management

5.3.1 Recommended Medication Protocols (Anticholinergic and Antihypertensive Agents)

Hemodynamic changes during ECT, although drastic, are mostly predictable. Several medications have been evaluated for their ability to ameliorate the hemodynamic alterations and reduce the risks associated with ECT. Anticholinergic agents are used to prevent bradycardia immediately after electrical stimulation. Intravenous atropine (0.4–0.8 mg) is effective in preventing the bradycardia [10, 57]. Previous studies demonstrated that intravenous administration of atropine several minutes before electrical stimulation is more reliable than intramuscular injection [58]. Glycopyrrolate (0.2–0.4 mg) is also effective in preventing bradycardia immediately after electrical stimulation [59]. When glycopyrrolate is used as the anticholinergic agent during ECT, tachycardia following the seizure is less common than when atropine is used.

The hyperdynamic state induced by sympathetic activation can be ameliorated by ganglion blockers [31], beta-blockers [60, 61], alpha-/beta-blockers [62, 63], alpha-2-agonists [64], Ca^{2+}-channel antagonists [65, 66], and nitrates [67, 68] (Table 5.3). Recent guidelines recommend the use of ultra-short-acting beta-blocker esmolol and the alpha-/beta-blocker labetalol, as antihypertensive medications for patients with cardiovascular complications [12, 59]. Ca^{2+}-channel antagonists, such as diltiazem [65] and nicardipine [66], are also effective for hemodynamic management during ECT. Nicardipine provokes temporary tachycardia because of its vasodilatory action. Glyceryl trinitrate [67, 68] and sodium nitroprusside [50] may be especially appropriate for use in patients with ischemic heart disease.

Some anesthetics can ameliorate the hemodynamic changes during ECT (Table 5.3). Hemodynamic alteration under propofol anesthesia is more stable than that under barbiturate anesthesia [69–71]. Additional use of sevoflurane has been proposed to blunt hemodynamic activation during ECT [72], although it requires a relatively long induction time and its use is associated with relatively short-duration ECT seizures.

Previous reports noted that several antihypertensive regimens, including use of esmolol or labetalol, are associated with relatively short seizure duration [73] (see Table 5.3). Use of propofol [74] and supplemental use of lidocaine [60] or sevoflurane [72] also decrease seizure duration. However, recent psychiatric studies demonstrated that seizure duration is not necessarily related to therapeutic efficacy [75]; only abortive or extremely short seizures (of less than 15 s) have limited utility [10]. Anesthesiologists should weigh the risks and benefits of antihypertensive regimens in their ECT management, especially for patients with cardiac or vascular complications.

5.3.2 Beta-Blockers

Administration of esmolol attenuates cardiovascular variations in the first 5 min after electrical stimulation. Although seizure duration may be affected with higher doses, esmolol appears to be effective in reducing the cardiovascular response to ECT [76, 77]. The recommended dose of esmolol for ECT is approximately $1\ \text{mg} \cdot \text{kg}^{-1}$ [10, 59].

With the use of labetalol, inconsistent effects on cardiovascular variations were found during the first few minutes after electrical stimulation, although the cardiovascular effects of the drug were significant after 5 min and thereafter; however, seizure duration was not studied in detail [62]. Further, although labetalol has been studied to a lesser extent than esmolol, it may have prolonged cardiovascular effects.

Landiolol is an ultra-short-acting, β1-selective, adrenergic receptor-blocking agent. It is rapidly hydrolyzed to an inactive form by both carboxylesterase in the liver and pseudocholinesterase in the plasma [78], resulting in an estimated half-life of about 4 min, which is significantly shorter than the elimination half-lives of conventional β1-blockers. In addition, landiolol hydrochloride is much more cardioselective ($\beta1/\beta2 = 255$) than currently available β1-blockers, such as esmolol hydrochloride ($\beta1/\beta2 = 33$) [78]. Landiolol effectively suppresses heart rate elevation after the electrical stimulation of ECT, although with inconsistent effects on arterial pressure [79, 80]. Saito et al. demonstrated that no change in HR was observed in patients who received landiolol $0.125\text{–}0.5\ \text{mg} \cdot \text{kg}^{-1}$ (Fig. 5.2) [79]. In one study, blood pressure increased after the electrical stimulation in both vehicle-treated and landiolol-treated groups, with no significant difference between the groups (Fig. 5.3). They also found that heart rate alteration was not observed in patients who received esmolol or landiolol (Fig. 5.4), whereas the effect of landiolol on blood pressure was minimal and less than that of esmolol (Fig. 5.5), and that cerebral blood flow velocity in the middle cerebral artery was not affected by the use of either esmolol or landiolol (Fig. 5.6). In another study, ECT seizure duration was unaffected by landiolol at $0.1\ \text{mg} \cdot \text{kg}^{-1}$ [81]. Furthermore, the echocardiographic study demonstrated that landiolol is a suitable agent to minimize systemic hemodynamic changes and transthoracic echocardiographic variability after ECT (Table 5.4) [82]. Hence, landiolol can be considered a suitable alternative to esmolol to attenuate the cardiovascular effects of ECT, although its effects on arterial blood pressure need further investigation.

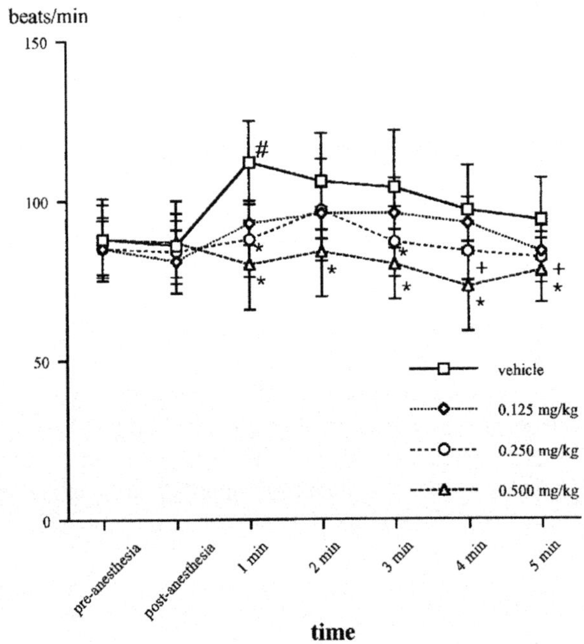

Fig. 5.2 Heart rate after the administration of landiolol. Heart rate increased 1 min after electrical stimulation in the vehicle-treated group (#$P < 0.01$). No change in heart rate was observed in patients who received landiolol 0.125–0.5 $mg \cdot kg^{-1}$. Patients who received 0.25–0.5 $mg \cdot kg^{-1}$ landiolol had lower mean heart rate values after electrical stimulation compared to patients who received vehicle (*$P < 0.01$ at 1–5 min after electrical stimulation in the patients who received 0.5 $mg \cdot kg^{-1}$ landiolol, *$P < 0.01$ at 1 and 3 min and +$P < 0.05$ at 4 and 5 min after stimulation in the patients who received 0.25 $mg \cdot kg^{-1}$ landiolol) (From Saito et al. [79]. Used with permission)

5.4 Respiratory Management

Although respiratory care during ECT is required for only approximately 10 min, inappropriate management interferes with the efficacy of the therapy and increases the risk of complications [10, 24, 83]. Following anesthesia induction with an anesthetic agent and a muscle relaxant, the airway should be secured and ventilation should be supported manually. Hypocarbia induced by hyperventilation may be required in some patients, to ensure appropriate seizure duration, because hypocarbia prolongs seizure duration [84, 85]. Our previous study [24] demonstrated that end-tidal carbon dioxide measurement at the nostrils is effective in maintaining the required carbon dioxide level before electrical stimulation. In some patients for whom mask ventilation is difficult because of oromandibular anatomic reasons, airway devices, including laryngeal masks, can be used for adequate ventilation [86]. Since incidents involving regurgitation are very rare, intubation is not necessary in most cases [87]. Some authors, however, recommend

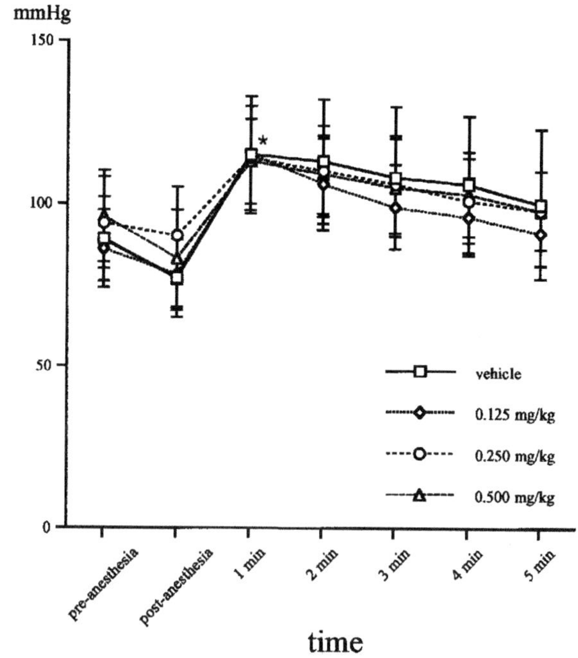

Fig. 5.3 Blood pressure after the administration of landiolol. Blood pressure increased at 1 min after stimulation in all groups ($P < 0.05$). There were no significant differences between the groups (From Saito et al. [79]. Used with permission)

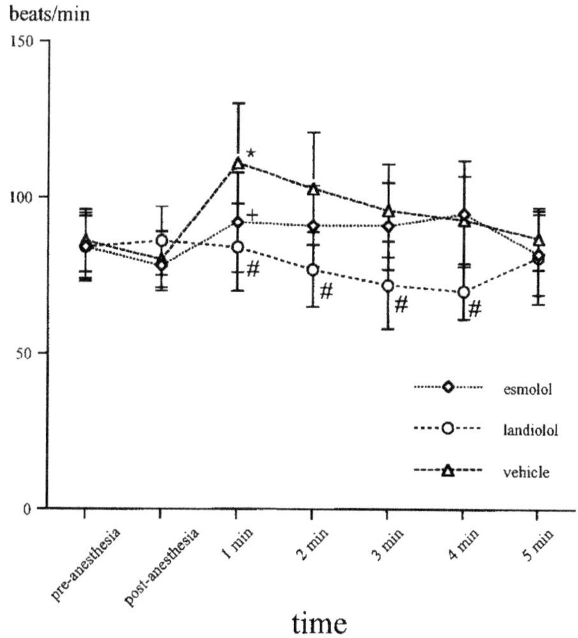

Fig. 5.4 Heart rate after the administration of esmolol or landiolol. Heart rate increased at 1 min after electrical stimulation in the vehicle-treated group as observed in Study 1 ($P < 0.01$). Heart rate alteration was not observed in the patients who received esmolol or landiolol. Patients who received esmolol had a significantly lower heart rate at 1 min after the stimulation compared to patients who received vehicle ($+P < 0.05$). Patients who received landiolol had lower heart rate values 1–4 min after the stimulation compared to patients who received vehicle ($*P < 0.01$) (From Saito et al. [79]. Used with permission)

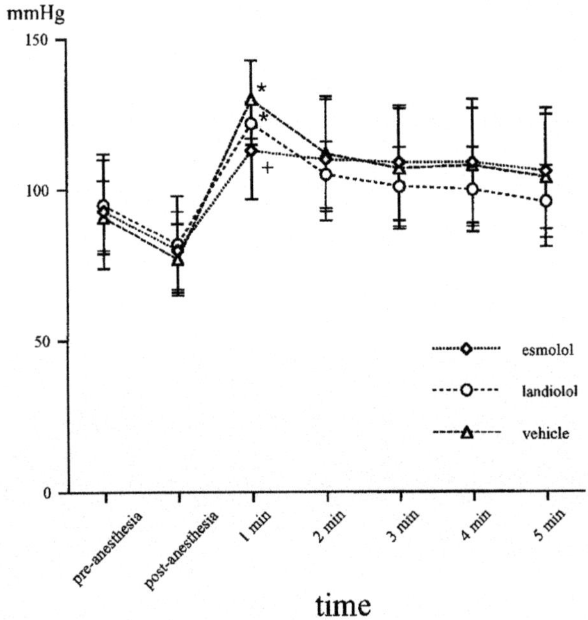

Fig. 5.5 Blood pressure after the administration of esmolol or landiolol. Blood pressure increased at 1 min after electrical stimulation in patients who received vehicle or landiolol (*$P < 0.01$). Blood pressure in the patients who received esmolol did not change after the stimulation and the value at 1 min after the stimulation was lower than the corresponding value in vehicle-treated patients (+$P < 0.01$) (From Saito et al. [79]. Used with permission)

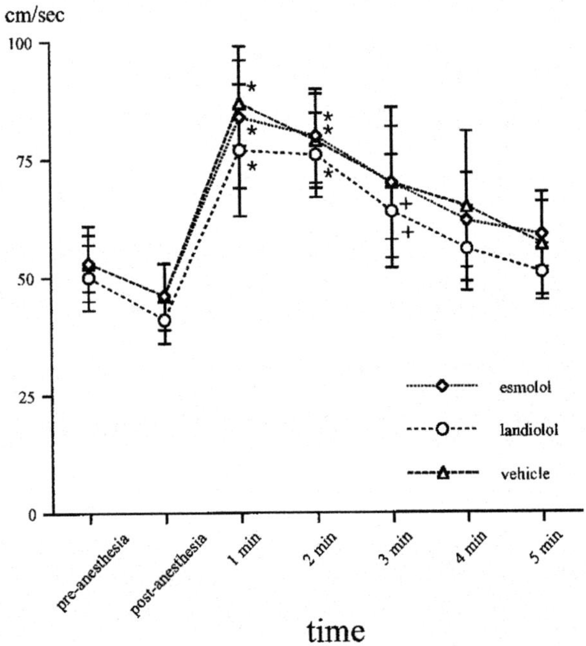

Fig. 5.6 Cerebral blood flow velocity after the administration of esmolol or landiolol. Mean cerebral blood flow velocity in the middle cerebral artery increased at 1–2 min after electrical stimulation in the vehicle-treated group (*$P < 0.01$). The value in the esmolol- or landiolol-treated group increased at 1–3 min after the stimulation (*$P < 0.01$ at 1–2 min after the stimulation, +$P < 0.05$ at 3 min after the stimulation). There were no significant differences between groups (From Saito et al. [79]. Used with permission)

Table 5.4 Time course of changes in hemodynamic variables in the two groups during electroconvulsive therapy (ECT)

Measurement time	1	2	3	4	5	6	7
Heart rate (beats/min)							
Control	77 ± 11	74 ± 9	100 ± 12*,#	96 ± 10*,#	93 ± 7*,#	76 ± 3	76 ± 8
Landiolol	75 ± 9	76 ± 7	78 ± 2	74 ± 4	76 ± 3	73 ± 5	73 ± 4
MAP (mmHg)							
Control	83 ± 6	78 ± 6	129 ± 10*,#	122 ± 10*,#	112 ± 8*,#	98 ± 4*,#	85 ± 6
Landiolol	84 ± 4	78 ± 6	111 ± 3*	109 ± 3*	93 ± 4	86 ± 3	86 ± 4
End-diastolic area (cm^2)							
Control	9.7 ± 0.9	10.0 ± 0.6	10.1 ± 0.8	9.7 ± 0.7	9.7 ± 0.4	9.7 ± 0.6	9.9 ± 0.3
Landiolol	9.8 ± 1.1	9.9 ± 1.0	10.0 ± 0.7	9.9 ± 0.6	9.8 ± 0.7	9.9 ± 0.7	9.7 ± 0.5
End-systolic area (cm^2)							
Control	4.9 ± 0.2	4.8 ± 0.2	6.1 ± 0.1*,#	6.1 ± 0.2*,#	5.7 ± 0.2*,#	5.1 ± 0.2	4.9 ± 0.2
Landiolol	5.0 ± 0.2	4.8 ± 0.3	5.2 ± 0.3	5.0 ± 0.2	5.0 ± 0.2	4.8 ± 0.2	4.9 ± 0.2
Fractional area change (%)							
Control	48 ± 3	51 ± 4	38 ± 4*,#	36 ± 4*,#	40 ± 3*,#	47 ± 3	50 ± 1
Landiolol	47 ± 7	50 ± 6	47 ± 4	48 ± 3	48 ± 4	50 ± 4	48 ± 3
Systolic BP/EDA-ESA ($mmHg/cm^2$)							
Control	22 ± 3	19 ± 2	38 ± 6*,#	41 ± 8*,#	33 ± 4*,#	26 ± 3	21 ± 2
Landiolol	23 ± 7	20 ± 4	27 ± 3	26 ± 3	24 ± 3	21 ± 3	22 ± 3

From Ide et al. [82]. Used with permission

Values are expressed as mean ± standard deviation

*$P < 0.05$ compared with period 1, #$P < 0.05$ compared with landiolol group

MAP mean arterial pressure, *EDA* end-diastolic area, *ESA* end-systolic area, *BP* blood pressure

1 awake, *2* 1 min after thiopental administration, *3* 1 min after electrical shock, *4* 2 min after electrical shock, *5* 3 min after electrical shock, *6* 5 min after electrical shock, and *7* 10 min after electrical shock

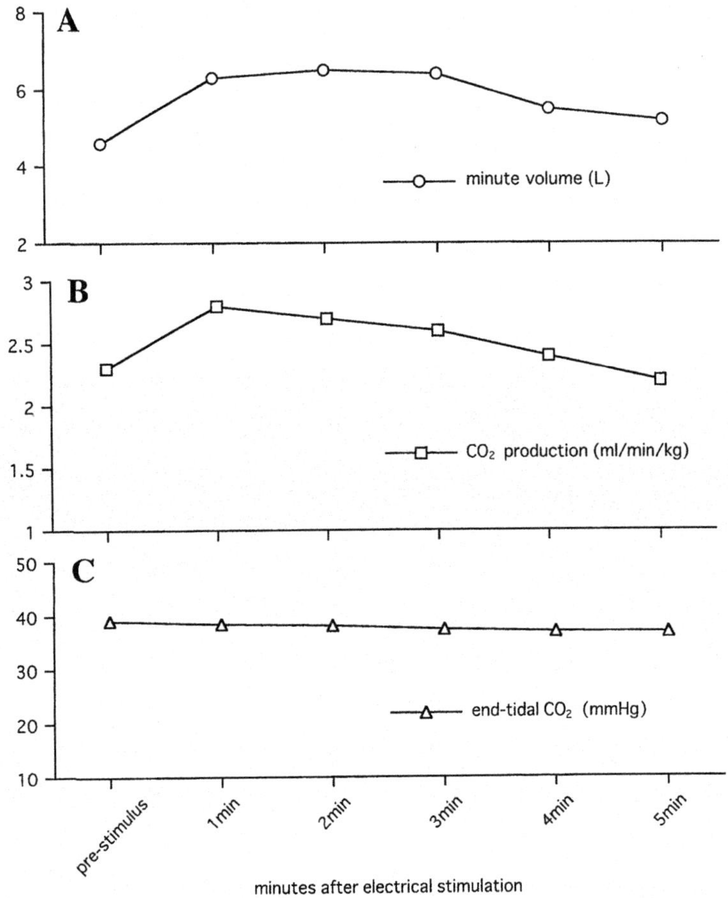

Fig. 5.7 Typical respiratory management during electroconvulsive therapy (ECT) in a patient. (**a**) Minute volume trend when the anesthetist tried to maintain the end-tidal carbon dioxide partial pressure at 35–40 mmHg. (**b**) Typical trend of carbon dioxide production during ECT. (**c**) End-tidal carbon dioxide partial pressure trend when expired air was sampled from the laryngeal mask airway and the anesthetist tried to maintain the end-tidal carbon dioxide partial pressure at 35–40 mmHg (From Saito et al. [15]. Used with permission)

intubation during ECT when this therapy is applied for depression during late pregnancy [88, 89].

During electrical stimulation, even under the use of a muscle relaxant, the facial muscles are electrically stimulated. Dental and lingual protection should be used, either by the use of a specially designed mouthpiece or by fixing the mandibular joint at the maximally closed position [10].

After completion of the electrical stimulation, oxygen consumption and carbon dioxide production are elevated by the seizure activity [46] (Fig. 5.7). Fasciculation that is induced by succinylcholine also contributes to the elevated oxygen demand

and carbon dioxide production [24]. To overcome the elevated oxygen demand and carbon dioxide production, anesthesiologists should increase ventilation volume adequately. Hypoxia and/or hypercarbia induced by inadequate ventilation after the electrical stimulation aggravate hypertension and tachycardia after the seizure [24]. The incidence and intensity of postictal excitement and headache may also be increased by prolonged hypercarbia [86].

5.5 Conclusion

ECT is a unique therapy that intentionally provokes seizures by applying an electrical current to the human central nervous system. In general, seizures are believed to be detrimental to the nervous system, and it is recommended that they be suppressed as early as possible. This general concept may be the main reason for public resistance to this therapy. However, the clinical effectiveness of this therapy for several types of psychiatric disorders overcomes the opposition to its application and promotes its clinical use worldwide. Safe physical management by anesthesiologists greatly contributes to the safety of ECT under muscle relaxation. To maintain social confidence and to refine the therapy, anesthesiologists should play an essential role in both clinical activities and laboratory research related to ECT.

References

1. Ishihara K, Sasa M. Mechanism underlying the therapeutic effects of electroconvulsive therapy (ECT) on depression. Jpn J Pharmacol. 1999;80:185–9.
2. Wahlund B, von Rosen D. ECT of major depressed patients in relation to biological and clinical variables: a brief overview. Neuropsychopharmacology. 2003;28:S21–6.
3. Fink M. Convulsive therapy: a review of the first 55 years. J Affect Disord. 2001;63:1–15.
4. Philibert RA, Richards L, Lynch CF, Winokur G. Effect of ECT on mortality and clinical outcome in geriatric unipolar depression. J Clin Psychiatry. 1995;56:390–4.
5. UK ECT Review Group. Efficacy and safety of electroconvulsive therapy in depressive disorders: a systematic review and meta-analysis. Lancet. 2003;361:799–808.
6. Selvin BL. Electroconvulsive therapy—1987. Anesthesiology. 1987;67:367–85.
7. Kramer BA. Use of ECT in California, 1977–1983. Am J Psychiatry. 1985;142:1190–2.
8. Abrams R. Electroconvulsive therapy. New York: Oxford University Press; 1988.
9. Duffett R, Lelliott P. Auditing electroconvulsive therapy. The third cycle. Br J Psychiatry. 1998;172:401–5.
10. Weiner RD, Coffey CE, Fochtmann LJ, editors. The practice of electroconvulsive therapy; recommendations for treatment, training and privileging. 2nd ed. Washington, DC: American Psychiatric Association; 2001.
11. Simpson KH, Lynch L. Anesthesia and electroconvulsive therapy. Anesthesia. 1998;53:615–7.
12. Gaines III GY, Rees DI. Anesthetic considerations for electroconvulsive therapy. South Med J. 1992;85:469–82.
13. Jones RM, Knight PR. Cardiovascular and humoral responses to electroconvulsive therapy. Anesthesia. 1981;36:795–9.

14. Weigner MB, Partridge BL, Hauger R. Prevention of the cardiovascular and neuroendocrine response to electroconvulsive therapy. II. Effects of pretreatment regimens on catecholamines, ACTH, vasopressin, and cortisol. Anesth Analg. 1991;73:563–9.
15. Saito S. Anesthesia management for electroconvulsive therapy: hemodynamic and respiratory management. J Anesth. 2005;19:142–9.
16. Morley JE, Silver AJ. Nutritional issues in nursing home care. Ann Intern Med. 1995;123:850–9.
17. Harter RL. Intravenous anesthetics. In: White PF, editor. Anesthesia drug manual. Philadelphia: Saunders; 1996. p. 252–8.
18. Mokriski BK, Nagle SE, Papuchis GC, Cohen SM, Waxman GJ. Electroconvulsive therapy-induced cardiac arrhythmias during anesthesia with methohexital, thiamylal, or thiopental sodium. J Clin Anesth. 1992;4:208–12.
19. Decina P, Malitz S, Sackeim HA, Holzer J, Yudofsky S. Cardiac arrest during ECT modified by beta-adrenergic blockade. Am J Psychiatry. 1984;141:298–300.
20. Liebowitz NR, el-Mallakh RS. Cardiac arrest during ECT: a cholinergic phenomenon? J Clin Psychiatry. 1993;54:279–80.
21. Gabrielli A, Layon AJ, Cole P, Holbert R, Modell JH. Prolonged cardiopulmonary resuscitation with preservation of cerebral function in an elderly patient with asystole after electroconvulsive therapy. J Clin Anesth. 2002;14:234–40.
22. Huuhka MJ, Seinela L, Reinikainen P, Leinonen EV. Cardiac arrhythmias induced by ECT in elderly psychiatric patients: experience with 48-hour Holter monitoring. J ECT. 2003;19:22–5.
23. Bergsholm P, Bleie H, Gran L, d'Elia G. Cardiovascular response and seizure duration as determined by electroencephalography during unilateral electroconvulsive therapy. Acta Psychiatr Scand. 1993;88:25–8.
24. Saito S, Kadoi Y, Nishihara F, Aso C, Goto F. End-tidal carbon dioxide monitoring stabilized hemodynamic changes during ECT. J ECT. 2003;19:26–30.
25. Swartz CM. Physiological response to ECT stimulus dose. Psychiatry Res. 2000;97:229–35.
26. Yanovski A, Kron RE, Townsend RR, Ford V. The clinical utility of ambulatory blood pressure and heart rate monitoring in psychiatric inpatients. Am J Hypertens. 1998;11:309–15.
27. Mann J, Manevitz AZ, Chen JS, Johnson KS, Adelsheimer EF, Azima-Heller R, Massina A, Wilner PJ. Acute effects of single and repeated electroconvulsive therapy on plasma catecholamines and blood pressure in major depressive disorder. Psychiatry Res. 1990;34:127–37.
28. Knos GB, Sung YF, Cooper RC, Stoudemire A. Electroconvulsive therapy-induced hemodynamic changes unmask unsuspected coronary artery disease. J Clin Anesth. 1990;2:37–41.
29. Nishihara F, Saito S, Tobe M, Harada N, Kadoi Y, Goto F. Hemodynamic changes during electroconvulsive therapy under propofol anesthesia. J Anesth. 2002;16:332–5.
30. Messina AG, Paranicas M, Katz B, Markowitz J, Yao FS, Devereux BB. Effect of electroconvulsive therapy on the electrocardiogram and echocardiogram. Anesth Analg. 1992;75:511–4.
31. Dolinski SY, Zvara DA. Anesthetic considerations of cardiovascular risk during electroconvulsive therapy. Convuls Ther. 1997;13:157–64.
32. Kadoi Y, Saito S, Seki S, Ide M, Morita T, Goto F. Electroconvulsive therapy impairs systolic performance of the left ventricle. Can J Anesth. 2001;48:405–8.
33. Kadoi Y, Saito S, Ide M, Toda H, Sekimoto K, Seki S, Takahashi K, Goto F. The comparative effects of propofol versus thiopentone on left ventricular function during electroconvulsive therapy. Anaesth Intensive Care. 2003;31:172–5.
34. Lopez-Gomez D, Sanchez-Corral MA, Cobo JV, Jara F, Esplugas E. Myocardial infarction after electroconvulsive therapy. Rev Esp Cardiol. 1999;52:536.
35. Ali PB, Tidmarsh MD. Cardiac rupture during electroconvulsive therapy. Anaesthesia. 1997;52:884–6.
36. Zielinski RJ, Roose SP, Devanand DP, Woodring S, Sackeim HA. Cardiovascular complications of ECT in depressed patients with cardiac disease. Am J Psychiatry. 1993;150:904–9.

37. Brodersen P, Paulson OB, Bolwig TG, Rogon ZE, Rafaelsen OJ, Lassen NA. Cerebral hyperemia in electrically induced epileptic seizures. Arch Neurol. 1973;28:334–8.
38. Saito S, Yoshikawa D, Nishihara F, Morita T, Kitani Y, Amaya T, Fujita T. The cerebral hemodynamic response to electrically induced seizures in man. Brain Res. 1995;673:93–100.
39. Saito S, Miyoshi S, Yoshikawa D, Shimada H, Morita T, Kitani Y. Regional cerebral oxygen saturation during electroconvulsive therapy: monitoring by near-infrared spectrophotometry. Anesth Analg. 1996;83:726–30.
40. Vollmer-Haase J, Folkerts HW, Haase CG, Deppe M, Ringelstein EB. Cerebral hemodynamics during electrically induced seizures. NeuroReport. 1998;9:407–10.
41. Fabbri F, Henry ME, Renshaw PF, Nadgir S, Ehrenberg BL, Franceschini MA, Fantini S. Bilateral near-infrared monitoring of the cerebral concentration and oxygen-saturation of hemoglobin during right unilateral electro-convulsive therapy. Brain Res. 2003;992:193–204.
42. Saito S, Kadoi Y, Iriuchijima N, Obata H, Arai K, Morita T, Goto F. Reduction of cerebral hyperemia with antihypertensive medication after electroconvulsive therapy. Can J Anaesth. 2000;47:767–74.
43. Saito S, Kadoi Y, Nara T, Sudo M, Obata H, Morita T, Goto F. The comparative effects of propofol versus thiopental on middle cerebral artery blood flow velocity during electroconvulsive therapy. Anesth Analg. 2000;91:1531–6.
44. Miller AL, Shamban AT, Corddry DH, Kiney CA. Cerebral metabolic responses to electroconvulsive shock and their modification by hypercapnia. J Neurochem. 1982;38:916–24.
45. Barkai AI, Prohovnik I, Young WL, Durkin M, Nelson HD. Alternations of local cerebral blood flow and glucose uptake by electroconvulsive shock in rats. Biol Psychiatry. 1991;30:269–82.
46. Szirmai I, Boldizsar F, Fisher J. Correlation between blood gases, glycolytic enzymes and EEG during electroconvulsive treatment in relaxation. Acta Psychiatr Scand. 1975;51:171–81.
47. Hsiao JK, Messenheimer JA, Evans DL. ECT and neurological disorders. Convuls Ther. 1987;3:121–36.
48. MacKenzie RA, Southorn PA, Stensrad PE. Anesthesia at remote locations. In: Miller RD, editor. Anesthesia. 5th ed. Philadelphia.: Churchill Livingstone; 2000. p. 2241–69.
49. Weisberg LA, Elliott D, Mielke D. Intracerebral hemorrhage following electroconvulsive therapy. Neurology. 1991;41:1849.
50. Viguera A, Rordorf G, Schouten R, Welch C, Drop LJ. Intracranial haemodynamics during attenuated responses to electroconvulsive therapy in the presence of an intracerebral aneurysm. J Neurol Neurosurg Psychiatry. 1998;64:802–5.
51. Kolano JW, Chhibber A, Calalang CC. Use of esmolol to control bleeding and heart rate during electroconvulsive therapy in a patient with an intracranial aneurysm. J Clin Anesth. 1997;9:493–5.
52. Ogawa-Okamoto C, Saito S, Nishihara F, Yuki N, Goto F. Blood pressure control with glyceryl trinitrate during electroconvulsive therapy in a patient with cerebral aneurysm. Eur J Anaesthesiol. 2003;20:70–8.
53. Salaris S, Szuba MP, Traber K. ECT and intracranial vascular masses. J ECT. 2000;16:198–203.
54. Hunt SA, Kaplan E. ECT in the presence of a cerebral aneurysm. J ECT. 1998;14:123–4.
55. Gardner MW, Kellner CH. Safe use of ECT with an intracranial aneurysm. J ECT. 1998;14:290–2.
56. Najjar F, Guttmacher LB. ECT in the presence of intracranial aneurysm. J ECT. 1998;14:266–71.
57. Kramer BA. Anticholinergics and ECT. Convuls Ther. 1993;9:293–300.
58. Kramer BA, Afrasiabi A, Pollock VE. Intravenous versus intramuscular atropine in ECT. Am J Psychiatry. 1992;149:1258–60.
59. Ding Z, White PF. Anesthesia for electroconvulsive therapy. Anesth Analg. 2002;94:1351–64.

60. Weinger MB, Partridge BL, Hauger R, Mirow A. Prevention of the cardiovascular and neuroendocrine response to electroconvulsive therapy: I. Effectiveness of pretreatment regimens on hemodynamics. Anesth Analg. 1991;13:556–62.
61. Howie MB, Hiestand DC, Zvara DA, Kim PY, McSweeney TD, Coffman JA. Defining the dose ranged for esmolol used in electroconvulsive therapy hemodynamic attenuation. Anesth Analg. 1992;75:805–10.
62. Castelli I, Steiner LA, Kaufmann MA, Alfille PH, Schouten R, Welch CA, Drop LJ. Comparative effects of esmolol and labetalol to attenuate hyperdynamic states after electroconvulsive therapy. Anesth Analg. 1995;80:557–61.
63. Stoudemire A, Knos G, Gladson M, Markwalter H, Sung YF, Morris R, Cooper R. Labetalol in the control of cardiovascular responses to electroconvulsive therapy in high-risk depressed medical patients. J Clin Psychiatry. 1990;51:508–12.
64. Fu W, Stool LA, White PF, Husain MM. Is oral clonidine effective in modifying the acute hemodynamic response during electroconvulsive therapy? Anesth Analg. 1998;86:1127–30.
65. Wajima Z, Yoshikawa T, Ogura A, Imanaga K, Shiga T, Inoue T, Ogawa R. The effects of diltiazem on hemodynamics and seizure duration during electroconvulsive therapy. Anesth Analg. 2001;92:1327–30.
66. Avramov MN, Stool LA, White PF, Husain MM. Effects of nicardipine and labetalol on the acute hemodynamic response to electroconvulsive therapy. J Clin Anesth. 1998;10:394–400.
67. Lee JT, Erbguth PH, Stevens WC, Sack RL. Modification of electroconvulsive therapy induced hypertension with nitroglycerin ointment. Anesthesiology. 1985;62:793–6.
68. Nurenberg JR. Intravenous nitroglycerine in the management of posttreatment hypertension during electroconvulsive therapy. J Nerv Ment Dis. 1991;179:291–4.
69. Rampton AJ, Griffin RM, Stuart CS, Durcan JJ, Huddy NC, Abbott MA. Comparison of methohexital and propofol for electroconvulsive therapy: effects on hemodynamic responses and seizure duration. Anesthesiology. 1989;70:412–7.
70. Fredman B, d'Etienne J, Smith I, Husain MM, White PF. Anesthesia for electroconvulsive therapy: effects of propofol and methohexital on seizure activity and recovery. Anesth Analg. 1994;79:75–9.
71. Boey WK, Lai FO. Comparison of propofol and thiopentone as anaesthetic agents for electroconvulsive therapy. Anaesthesia. 1990;45:623–8.
72. Wajima Z, Shiga T, Yoshikawa T, Ogura A, Inoue T, Ogawa R. Propofol alone, sevoflurane alone, and combined propofol-sevoflurane anaesthesia in electroconvulsive therapy. Anaesth Intensive Care. 2003;31:396–400.
73. van den Broek WW, Leentjens AFG, Mulder PGH, Kusuma A, Bruijn JA. Low-dose esmolol bolus reduces seizure duration during electroconvulsive therapy: a double-blind, placebo-controlled study. Br J Anaesth. 1999;83:271–4.
74. Simpson KH, Halsall PJ, Carr CME, Stewart KG. Propofol reduces seizure duration in patients having anaesthesia for electroconvulsive therapy. Br J Anaesth. 1988;61:343–4.
75. Lalla FR, Milroy T. The current status of seizure duration in the practice of electroconvulsive therapy. Can J Psychiatry. 1996;41:299–304.
76. Kovac AL, Goto H, Arakawa K, Pardo MP. Esmolol bolus and infusion attenuates increases in blood pressure and heart rate during electroconvulsive therapy. Can J Anaesth. 1990;37:58–62.
77. Zvara DA, Brooker RF, McCall WV, Foreman AS, Hewitt C, Murphy BA, Royster RL. The effect of esmolol on ST-segment depression and arrhythmias after electroconvulsive therapy. Convuls Ther. 1997;13:165–74.
78. Iguchi S, Iwamura H, Nishizaki M, Hayashi A, Senokuchi K, Kobayashi K, Sakaki K, Hachiya K, Ichioka Y, Kawamura M. Development of a highly cardioselective ultra short-acting beta-blocker, ONO-1101. Chem Pharm Bull. 1992;40:1462–9.
79. Saito S, Nishihara F, Akihiro T, Nishikawa K, Obata H, Goto F, Yuki N. Landiolol and esmolol prevent tachycardia without altering cerebral blood flow. Can J Anaesth. 2005;52:1027–34.

80. Nomoto K, Suzuki T, Serada K, Oe K, Yoshida T, Yamada S. Effects of landiolol on hemodynamic response and seizure duration during electroconvulsive therapy. J Anesth. 2006;20:183–7.
81. Sakamoto A, Ogawa R, Suzuki H, Kimura M, Okubo Y, Fujiya T. Landiolol attenuates acute hemodynamic responses but does not reduce seizure duration during maintenance electroconvulsive therapy. Psychiatry Clin Neurosci. 2004;58:630–5.
82. Ide M, Kadoi Y, Saito S, Takahashi K, Sawano Y, Miyazaki M, Shimada H. Effects of landiolol on left ventricular function during electroconvulsive therapy: a transthoracic echocardiographic study. J Anesth. 2010;24:272–6.
83. Zhu B, Ishida K, Oritani S, Fujita M, Maeda H, Tanaka T, Tanaka N. Sudden death following psychiatric electroconvulsive therapy: a case report. Jpn J Legal Med. 1998;52:149–52.
84. Chater SN, Simpson KH. Effect of passive hyperventilation on seizure duration in patients undergoing electroconvulsive therapy. Br J Anaesth. 1988;60:70–3.
85. Crawford CD, Butler P, Froese A. Arterial PaO2 and PaCO2 influence seizure duration in dogs receiving electroconvulsive therapy. Can J Anaesth. 1987;34:437–41.
86. Nishihara F, Ohkawa M, Hiraoka H, Yuki N, Saito S. Benefits of the laryngeal mask for airway management during electroconvulsive therapy. J ECT. 2003;19:211–6.
87. Kadar AG, Ing CH, White PF, Wakefield CA, Kramer BA, Clark K. Anesthesia for electroconvulsive therapy in obese patients. Anesth Analg. 2002;94:360–1.
88. Livingston JC, Johnstone Jr WM, Hadi HA. Electroconvulsive therapy in a twin pregnancy: a case report. Am J Perinatol. 1994;11:116–8.
89. Walker R, Swartz CM. Electroconvulsive therapy during high-risk pregnancy. Gen Hosp Psychiatry. 1994;16:348–53.

Postprocedural Assessments and Considerations

6

Masami Sato

Abstract

Postictal agitation is a frequent complication during the emergence period after ECT. This symptom commonly resolves naturally within 1 h, but a severe or persistent episode requires pharmacological treatment with benzodiazepines or propofol to control the acute situation. Hypoxemia following ECT can also occur in this period, and monitoring of oxygen saturation should be continued until psychomotor function resumes. When desaturation is prolonged, initial pulmonary aspiration of increased saliva or gastric contents is suggested. Patients generally require about 2 h of post-ECT care in the recovery room and adverse symptoms, especially headache, should be noted. Elderly patients have a high risk of fall and should be monitored carefully. Memory disturbance is an important cognitive impairment during and after ECT course and may impair optimal functioning. In some cases, ECT parameters should be modified based on the assessment of cognitive function to minimize this adverse effect. Continuation/maintenance ECT is an effective treatment option for relapse prevention after successful treatment with index ECT and is often performed in an ambulatory setting. The decision to transfer the patient from inpatient to ambulatory ECT requires careful assessment of the treatment response and adverse effects of ECT.

Keywords

Post-ECT recovery • Postictal agitation • Cognitive impairment • Ambulatory ECT • Continuation/maintenance ECT

M. Sato (✉)
Department of Anesthesia, Kyoto University Hospital, 54 Shogoin-Kawahara-cho, Sakyo-ku, Kyoto 606-8507, Japan
e-mail: masami@kb3.so-net.ne.jp

S. Saito (ed.), *Anesthesia Management for Electroconvulsive Therapy*,
DOI 10.1007/978-4-431-55717-3_6

6.1 Emergence Period

6.1.1 Neurological Management

6.1.1.1 Postictal Agitation

Cognitive impairment is the most notable and distressing complication of electroconvulsive therapy (ECT), with three types of cognitive impairment observed: postictal agitation, interictal confusion, and memory disturbance [1]. Postictal agitation is a relatively frequent adverse effect immediately after ECT, with reported rates of 7 %, 10 %, and up to 36 % of patients who undergo an ECT course [2–5] (Table 6.1). The clinical characteristics of postictal agitation include disorientation, motor restlessness, aimless movement, nonresponse to verbal commands, panic-like behavior, and even attempts to pull out intravenous lines and leave the recovery room, which may be a hazard to the patient and the staff in the recovery room. Delirious patients, especially the elderly, may also be at increased risk of falls. In ambulatory ECT, prolonged postictal agitation may delay recovery and result in unanticipated admission. Emergence of severe postictal agitation does not mandate cessation of the ECT course, but can lead to patients withdrawing their consent to the treatment. The cause of postictal delirium is thought to be the seizure itself. Postictal agitation lasts from 5 min to 1 h in the immediate postictal phase and resolves naturally over time. The symptom initially appears to be agitation, but may rarely be nonconvulsive epileptic activity. Therefore, an electroencephalography (EEG) trace needs to be examined to rule out prolonged seizures as a cause of postictal agitation.

Prophylaxis and Treatment of Postictal Agitation

The severity of postictal agitation ranges from mild and self-limiting to severe. If the environment permits or the degree of agitation is mild, nonpharmacological interventions such as the brief use of restraints and maintenance of intravenous access can be effective as primary care to ensure patient safety and permit efficient pharmacological treatment. If supportive treatment is unsuccessful or the degree of agitation is severe and persistent, intravenous pharmacological treatment should be started to control the acute situation, along with subsequent prophylactic measures at future sessions, including provision of sufficient time and caregivers, because postictal agitation tends to recur in the same patient [3].

The standard pharmacological treatment for both postictal agitation and prolonged seizure is administration of intravenous benzodiazepines such as midazolam, lorazepam, and diazepam. Midazolam is short-acting and thus is most commonly used for these purposes at a dose of 0.5–2 mg [6]. Other effective treatments include intravenous antipsychotic medications, with intravenous haloperidol 5–20 mg being a good second option. Propofol and methohexital are also effective for postictal agitation and have the advantage of being immediately at hand if they are used as an anesthetic agent. The effective dose of methohexital for postictal agitation is usually half of the dose used for the induction of anesthesia [3]. Administration of propofol provides good control of postictal agitation as either

Table 6.1 Patient characteristics and recovery profiles in the PACU in ambulatory ECT (762 ECT procedures of 40 patients) (Revised from Ref. [5])

Age (year)		56 ± 16
Sex (male/female)		17/23
ASA physical status (1/2/3)		0/35/5
Diagnosis	Mood disorder	27
	Schizophrenia	10
	Psychiatric disorder by psychogenesis substance	2
	Dystonia	1
Anesthetic agents	Propofol	720 (95 %, 39 patients)
	Thiopental	33 (4 %, 1 patient)
	Sevoflurane	9 (1 %, 2 patients)
Muscle relaxant	Succinylcholine	762 (100 %, 40 patients)
Time from PACU admission until	Fluid intake (min)	55 ± 27
	Walking (min)	70 ± 29
	Voiding (min)	82 ± 29
	Discharge (min)	110 ± 38
Total DSU stay time[a] (min)		172 ± 38
Unplanned hospital admission		0
Adverse events	Agitation	54 (7 %, 11 patients)
	Headache	39 (5 %, 11 patients)
	Nausea	4 (0.5 %, 4 patients)
	Vomiting	0
Medication	Oxygen[b]	161 (21 %, 10 patients)
	Sedative agent	25 (3 %, 6 patients)
	Analgesic agent	25 (3 %, 8 patients)
	Cardiovascular agent[c]	2 (0.3 %, 1 patient)
	Antiemetic agent	1 (0.1 %, 1 patient)

Values are shown as mean ± SD, patient number, or number of ECT procedures (%, patient number)

PACU postanesthesia care unit, *ASA* American Society of Anesthesiologists, *DSU* Day Surgery Unit

[a]Time to discharge from arrival at DSU

[b]Oxygen was administered when SpO_2 was <90% without oxygen supplementation

[c]Administration of landiolol required for tachycardia

a bolus or a bolus followed by an infusion. The initial report of the effect of propofol in preventing postictal agitation by Augoustides et al. [7] dates back to 2002. The same group then reported successful use of propofol in management of 10 patients with severe and treatment-resistant postictal agitation in ECT, despite a prior inadequate response to intravenous midazolam and other agents [8]. In their reports, propofol in boluses of 0.1–2 mg/kg initially after seizure, followed by an infusion at 1.5–9 mg/kg/h for 20 min to 2 h, if needed, is effective for resistant cases of agitation. The safe use of propofol infusion requires monitoring of oxygen saturation of peripheral artery (SpO_2) and blood pressure to maintain the airway and avoid hypotension. A single bolus of propofol 0.5 mg/kg preemptively administered after the end of a seizure in 13 patients with a history of severe postictal agitation reduced the incidence of postictal agitation [9]. Patients and staff in a postanesthesia care unit (PACU) rated the emergence period as better in patients treated with propofol, although the time from the end of EEG seizure to transfer to the PACU was longer.

Dexmedetomidine, an α_2-adrenergic agonist, was first used in the context of ECT in an attempt to blunt the acute hemodynamic response to ECT and was also found to attenuate postictal agitation when given as premedication [10] or immediately after seizure conclusion [11, 12]. Premedication with intravenous dexmedetomidine 0.5 μg/kg 10 min before induction of anesthesia reduced the agitation score at 10 and 15 min after ECT in 15 patients who experienced severe postictal agitation, without shortening the duration of convulsion because of the lower dose of propofol used for anesthetic induction nor hypoxemia [10]. O'Brien et al. [11] and Bryson et al. [12] described the successful use of dexmedetomidine at 1 μg/kg for 10 min immediately after seizure conclusion in postictal management of severe agitation that was unresponsive to midazolam, ketamine, propofol, and olanzapine, although routine use of dexmedetomidine in ECT is not recommended because of its cost. Promethazine 25–50 mg orally given 1–2 h before each ECT session as an oral prophylaxis has also been proposed for postictal agitation in a case series of eight patients [13].

Factors Involved in Postictal Agitation

ECT technique and anesthetic and psychiatric factors, such as stimulus waveforms, electrode placement, concomitant lithium use, dosing of anesthetic agent and muscle relaxant, and high pre-ECT anxiety levels, have been implicated in onset of postictal agitation [3, 7, 14, 15]. Excess energy delivered to patients as a result of the gradual rise and offset of intensity in the sine wave stimulus results in adverse cardiovascular and cognitive effects, including postictal agitation. There is no significant difference on treatment efficiency using sine wave stimulation with brief pulse treatment, and thus brief pulse waveforms with less adverse cognitive effects have become the more commonly used stimulus. This shift in technique has resulted in a reduction in the intensity of cognitive side effects. Since bilateral electrode placement is more commonly associated with cognitive impairment, including postictal agitation, switching to a unilateral placement may reduce postictal agitation, if this change is clinically possible. Strongly left-handed patients presenting with postictal agitation after receiving right unilateral ECT may improve when switched to contralateral placement in order to stimulate the nondominant hemisphere. Since lithium has been associated with prolonged or severe postictal agitation, concomitant lithium therapy must be prophylactically discontinued or given at a minimum dose for 24 h before each ECT to reduce the incidence of postictal agitation [14].

Anesthetic contributory factors also have been addressed. Regarding muscle relaxants, Auriacombe et al. and Swartz suggested that increasing the dose of succinylcholine may reduce postictal agitation by reducing the release of lactate from muscle through minimizing muscular activity [2, 16]. Furthermore, insufficient doses of the induction agent have also been linked to postictal agitation, since this has been prevented in some cases by increasing the dose of methohexital in the ECT course within the range recommended clinically to maintain the seizure duration required for treatment [17]. Thus, possible anesthetic approaches to minimize postictal agitation after ECT include selection of appropriate dosages of anesthetic induction agents and muscle relaxants [7].

Predictors of postictal agitation also include patient and ECT variables. In 96 consecutive patients after the first ECT, Reti et al. found that the average seizure length for patients with postictal agitation was significantly longer than that for patients without agitation (86 vs. 59 s) [18], a long ECT seizure duration increased the likelihood of agitation, and patients with a seizure ≥80 s were very likely to be delirious in the PACU. As soon as therapeutic adequacy of the induced seizure is obtained during the seizure in patients with a tendency of postictal agitation, administration of benzodiazepines or anesthetic agents to terminate seizure can be recommended before seizure is prolonged. In a study of 50 patients, Kikuchi et al. found that postictal agitation occurred significantly more often in patients with catatonic features (88 %) compared to those without catatonic features (24 %) regardless of diagnosis [4]. The symptoms of postictal agitation were treated successfully with a propofol bolus, the same dose as the induction dosage or continuous infusion of propofol (4–8 mg/kg/h) for 15–20 min, and most postictal agitation after ECT improved with remission of catatonic symptoms. Age can be a risk factor for delirium in some settings: children after sevoflurane anesthesia are at high risk of emergence agitation, and elderly patients tend to be delirious in an intensive care unit. However, age was not found to be a significant factor for the development of postictal agitation in the ECT settings in the above studies [4, 18].

6.1.1.2 Persistent Seizure Activity

Persistent seizure activity (prolonged seizures and status epilepticus) or recurrence of seizure activity may occur after ECT in rare instances. Prolonged seizure activity is defined as a seizure lasting longer than 3 min with motor or EEG manifestations with reported rates of 1–2 % [3, 19]. Routine EEG monitoring is especially useful for the detection of prolonged seizures, because most seizures are undetectable by observation of motor activity alone. Young patients have lower seizure thresholds and a higher frequency of prolonged seizures [20]. Prolonged seizures are particularly likely to occur in the following circumstances: (1) at the first treatment, (2) during withdrawal of benzodiazepines, (3) in patients in whom proconvulsant medications (caffeine, theophylline) and lithium are used concurrently, and (4) in patients with epilepsy or preexisting paroxysmal EEG activity [21]. Prolonged seizures may result in an increased risk of postictal agitation and amnesia [18], and early recognition and treatment are particularly important for patients receiving ECT on an outpatient basis to prevent progression of seizures into status epilepticus, with resultant increases in morbidity and mortality. For patients with long seizures, switching to propofol anesthesia may be advantageous because seizures in ECT induced by propofol are significantly shorter than those with methohexital or thiopental [20]. The degree of shortening of seizures is also dependent on the dose of anesthetic agent [22], and increasing the anesthetic dose can also shorten the seizure duration in such patients keeping the recommended seizure duration for treatment.

Prolonged seizure can be terminated by intravenous administration of short-acting benzodiazepines (e.g., 1–2 mg midazolam) or a repeat dose of the anesthetic agent (e.g., methohexital or propofol). The dose should be repeated if seizure activity continues for 2 more minutes after pharmacological treatment. For continued epileptic activity, lorazepam (2–4 mg intravenously over 1 min) or diazepam (5–10 mg iv) and/or phenytoin (18–20 mg/kg) should be given. Immediate neurology consultation and checking of arterial blood gases and electrolytes are necessary if status epilepticus is suspected. An algorithm for management of prolonged seizure is shown in Fig. 6.1. Maintenance of adequate oxygenation is important during prolonged seizure and may be accomplished via positive-pressure

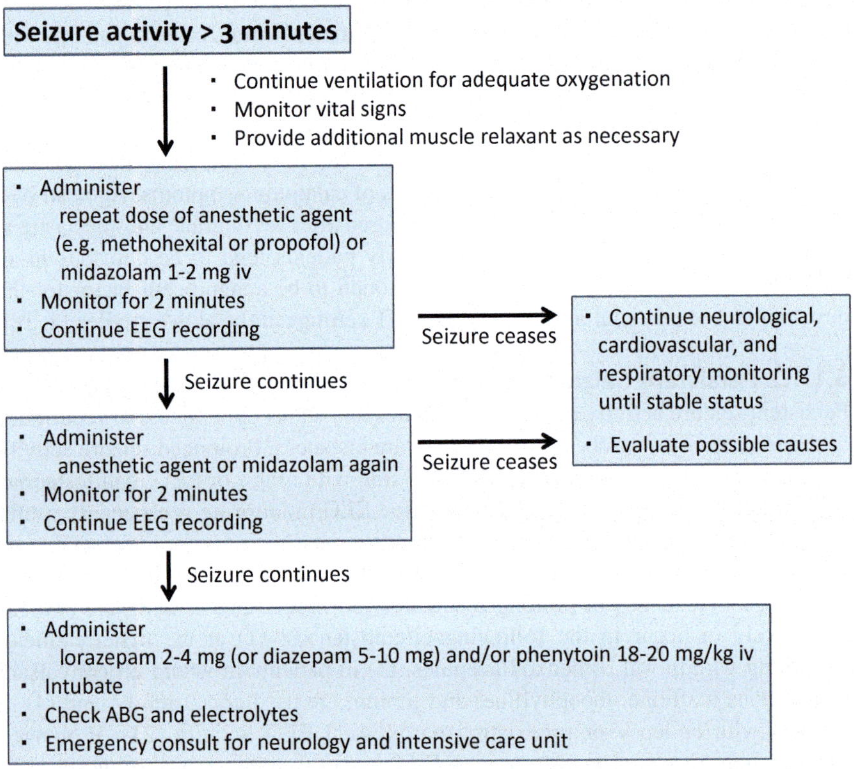

Fig. 6.1 Algorithm for management of prolonged seizures. *iv* intravenous, *EEG* electroencephalogram, *ABG* arterial blood gas

ventilation using a bag-mask or endotracheal tube if seizure activity is grossly prolonged (more than 5–10 min) or the patient becomes hypoxic. Vital signs (blood pressure, SpO_2, and electrocardiogram (ECG)) should be monitored continuously, and an additional dose of muscle relaxant should be provided as needed.

Status epilepticus is a life-threatening emergency and treatment should be started within 10 min of onset. Seizure activity that persists longer than 30 min results in greater morbidity (e.g., hyperthermia, circulatory collapse, and hypoxic encephalopathy) and mortality [23]. Lorazepam is more effective than phenobarbital or phenytoin, and lorazepam (0.1 mg/kg) is widely used for rapid seizure control with addition of phenytoin (18–20 mg/kg). Phenobarbital (20 mg/kg) is used as second-line treatment with assisted ventilation. Prolonged seizures and status epilepticus do not absolutely preclude further ECT. Concurrent use of an anticonvulsant agent may be indicated in some cases to prevent a further status epilepticus episode after ECT.

6.1.2 Respiratory Management

6.1.2.1 Postictal Respiratory Status

To secure the airway during ECT, most patients are manually ventilated with 100 % oxygen using a face mask with a standard circle system. Succinylcholine is commonly used as a muscle relaxant in ECT because of its short action. After completion of electrical stimulation, oxygen consumption and carbon dioxide production are elevated by the seizure activity [24]. Fasciculation induced by succinylcholine also contributes to this change. To overcome the elevated oxygen demand and carbon dioxide production, anesthesiologists should increase the ventilation volume adequately 5 min after electrical stimulation, and appropriate assisted ventilation should be continued until the effect of muscle relaxants disappear and spontaneous regular respiration resumes. Inadequate ventilation after electrical stimulation induces hypoxia or hypercarbia and results in hypertension and tachycardia after seizure [25]. Resuscitative equipment, including a laryngoscope, tracheal tube, laryngeal mask airway, and oral/nasal airway, should be available for the management of an airway emergency during ECT and the emergence period. A suction device should also be available to protect the airway from increased salivation induced by parasympathetic stimulation during ECT, since excessive saliva can induce laryngospasm, bronchospasm, pulmonary atelectasis, aspiration pneumonia, or negative pressure pulmonary edema. Routine administration of an anticholinergic agent such as glycopyrrolate or atropine before ECT to limit bradycardia and oral salivation depends on the condition of each patient [26]. Some patients who have experienced excessive oral secretion during ECT may need preventive administration of an anticholinergic agent to protect against pulmonary complications, although these agents can also induce tachycardia [27]. Glycopyrrolate (0.1–0.3 mg iv) is a better choice than atropine for the reduction of secretion because it is associated with less post-ECT tachycardia. In a review of respiratory complications in 75 patients during 612 ECT procedures, Tecoult et al. [28] identified one patient with potentially life-threatening aspiration pneumonia linked to inhalation of saliva. There were five episodes of severe laryngospasm and two of bronchospasm, among which four were induced by saliva.

The incidence of patients with $SpO_2 < 90\ \%$ without oxygen supplementation in the recovery room is 17 and 21 % [5, 29] (Table 6.1). SpO_2 during the emergence period is significantly lower than the preoperative value, and the lowest mean SpO_2 occurs at 4 min after arrival in the recovery room [29]. Since the main cause of postanesthesia hypoxemia after ECT is delay of psychomotor function recovery following convulsion, hypoxemia usually improves along with the recovery of psychomotor function. When hypoxemia continues after patients are fully awake after ECT without serious respiratory symptoms, a chest radiograph should be recorded with initial suspicion of pulmonary atelectasis. Inhalation of increased saliva is one cause of pulmonary atelectasis or pulmonary aspiration. In 12 patients undergoing ECT in whom chest radiographs were taken before and after ECT, Wayne et al. [30] found two cases with pulmonary atelectasis of the lower left lobe and one with subclinical pulmonary edema, despite these three patients having no clinical respiratory symptoms. Thus, the incidence of pulmonary atelectasis may be underestimated because patients may not show clinical symptoms and routine chest radiography is not performed, especially in confused patients. Since severe respiratory complications may be covered by hypoxemia, as discussed below, routine monitoring of SpO_2 is required, and an oxygen inhalation system should be available during the emergence and recovery periods.

6.1.2.2 Pulmonary Aspiration

Pulmonary aspiration following ECT was not uncommon before the use of muscle relaxants. The incidence has been reduced by introduction of muscle relaxants, but morbidity and mortality are relatively high in cases with severe pulmonary aspiration. Kurnutala et al. described the case of a 51-year-old man with depression who produced copious amounts of semisolid food and secretions through the mouth and nose just after convulsion and died of sepsis and multiorgan failure, despite taking nothing by mouth for approximately 14 h before ECT [31]. Burke et al. found two cases of aspiration pneumonia among 136 elderly patients receiving ECT [32]. Antacid premedication, application of cricoid pressure, and administration of ECT in a sitting position are simple methods to prevent pulmonary aspiration with few side effects [28]. Endotracheal intubation with cricoid pressure is the most effective approach, but elective tracheal intubation is rare, except for patients with a full stomach due to late pregnancy, severe obesity, or ileus. The major approach for preventing pulmonary aspiration, other than administration of an anticholinergic agent to reduce salivation, is following nothing per os (NPO) instructions before each ECT, especially for patients at higher risk of aspiration. Bedridden patients with severe psychiatric disease who need enteral tube feeding are also at high risk of retention of gastric contents.

6.1.2.3 Pulmonary Edema

Neurogenic or negative pressure pulmonary edema is an uncommon but potentially life-threatening respiratory complication following ECT. The severity of pulmonary edema after ECT varies from death to a requirement for oxygen administration. Buisseret described the first case of a 44-year-old woman who developed neurogenic pulmonary edema with difficulty breathing 1 h after ECT and eventually died of cardiopulmonary arrest 16 h after ECT [33]. Takahashi et al. reported the case of 47-year-old-man with depression, who developed acute dyspnea, hypoxemia, and mild hemoptysis 30 min after ECT. The patient was diagnosed with neurogenic pulmonary edema and needed oxygen inhalation for 2 days after ECT without requiring mechanical ventilation [34].

Production of negative pressure pulmonary edema after ECT requires the presence of a strong spontaneous inspiratory effort due to upper airway obstruction. Myers et al. described the case of a 21-year-old man who developed negative pressure pulmonary edema when spontaneous breathing had begun to return after his 28th ECT [35]. In this case, negative pressure pulmonary edema was probably precipitated by a large inspiratory effort due to inadequate muscular paralysis after termination of the seizure, either against a closed glottis or an airway obstructed by the bite block pushing the tongue into the posterior oropharyngeal space. Cochran et al. reported the case of 46-year-old woman who exhibited upper airway obstruction on awakening from her fourth ECT due to excess secretion that resulted in laryngospasm followed by negative pressure pulmonary edema [36]. Thus, it is important to prevent airway obstruction by excessive saliva or the bite block during emergence from anesthesia and to assist the smooth return of spontaneous respirations along with bag and mask ventilation. Since most patients do not develop pulmonary edema after their first ECT, its occurrence after ECT is difficult to predict. When respiratory symptoms such as hypoxemia and frothy pink sputum develop after ECT, pulmonary edema should be suspected and chest radiography is crucial for diagnosis. Pulmonary edema is treated in a supportive and conservative fashion, since most cases resolve within several days.

6.1.2.4 Pulmonary Embolism

Pulmonary embolism as a complication of ECT is rare and may be fatal. Weber et al. reported the case of a 59-year-old man who died 2 h after his second ECT because of emboli in both main branches of the pulmonary arteries [37]. The patient's inactivity due to his psychiatric status was likely to have resulted in a high degree of peripheral venous stasis. Mamah et al. described a 50-year-old man treated without anticoagulant therapy, who developed symptoms of pulmonary embolism such as chest tightness and hemoptysis immediately upon awakening from his eighth ECT in his fourth ECT course, with the condition later confirmed by computed tomography (CT) as pulmonary embolism [38]. The patient started continuous intravenous heparin infusion and his vital signs improved on the second day of infusion. The risk for venous thrombosis in this patient was prolonged inactivity, primarily due to depression, obesity, and diabetes. Both reports suggest that muscle contractions elicited during generalized seizure can dislodge a clot from a peripheral source, despite the use of succinylcholine.

Pulmonary embolism is also associated with respiratory distress, hypoxemia, and hemoptysis, and thus distinguishing this condition from pulmonary edema is sometimes difficult. Echocardiography, contrast CT, and pulmonary scintigraphy are recommended for patients with suspicious symptoms following seizures, and particularly in cases with a high risk of embolization. There is also a need to screen patients undergoing ECT for possible mechanical or pharmacological prophylaxis against pulmonary embolism [39]. This is especially true for patients who are bedridden or under restraint because of psychiatric disease, or those with cardiac risk factors or a history of deep venous thrombus/pulmonary embolism. Therapy for anticoagulation can be continued during ECT course to maintain an international normalized ratio (INR) of up to 3.5, unless there is an increased risk of intracranial hemorrhage. In a study with 33 patients receiving long-term warfarin therapy with INR <3.5, there were no ECT-related complications due to anticoagulation, such as intracerebral hemorrhage [40]. ECT can be considered in patients with a history of recent deep venous thrombus or pulmonary embolism, based on cardiopulmonary risk and the benefit of ECT for psychiatric stabilization [39].

6.1.3 Cardiovascular Management

Acute cardiovascular responses to ECT involve the sympathetic and parasympathetic branches of the autonomic nervous system. Between the electrical stimulus and the onset of seizure, bradycardia or asystole induced by vagal tone stimulation may last for more than 5 s. After onset of seizure, catecholamine surge induces significant tachycardia, hypertension, and sometimes arrhythmias. Some patients need antihypertensive drugs, β-blockers, or antiarrhythmic drugs to reduce these cardiovascular responses during ECT, but most hemodynamic changes resolve after the patient awakes. Mean blood pressure and heart rate are increased after electrical stimulation, reach maximum values approximately 1 min after stimulation, continue at this level for about 5 min, and return to baseline within 10 min [41]. Only 0.3 % of ambulatory ECT procedures require cardiovascular drugs (landiolol for tachycardia) in the PACU, and cardiovascular complications are not a source of recovery delay or unanticipated admission (Table 6.1). Although transient in nature, hemodynamic responses to ECT may occasionally extend beyond the expected recovery period and may lead to more serious outcomes in susceptible patients, including myocardial infarction, circulatory collapse, and atrial and ventricular arrhythmias [24].

Preexisting cardiac disease or cerebrovascular disease (e.g. cerebral aneurysms) are risk factors for increased complication rates and require tight hemodynamic control during the ECT and recovery periods [42]. Patients with such diseases should be encouraged to take all chronic cardiovascular medicines before ECT and sometimes need preventive administration of antihypertensive drugs or β-blockers before electrical stimulus to attenuate the hemodynamic response, although this requires caution because some of these drugs can produce adverse effects on the duration of the ECT-induced seizure activity [27]. Careful observation including ECG and routine monitoring of SpO_2 and noninvasive blood pressure must be done in the emergence and recovery periods for a patient with extensive circulation changes during ECT and a high risk of cardiovascular disease. Cardiovascular drugs to control postprocedural arrhythmia, tachycardia, and hypertension should also be available.

6.1.4 Effects of Anesthetic Agents on Emergence and Recovery Times

Emergence and recovery times are influenced directly by the choice of anesthetic agent and indirectly by the induced seizure being modified by the agent. Recently, ECT has become an ambulatory procedure for more patients, and this has made the times to emergence and to discharge from the PACU into the important outcomes, which are influenced by anesthetic agents. Although seizure duration is shorter with propofol than with other anesthetics (etomidate, methohexital, or thiopental), propofol has advantages of earlier recovery of orientation, general functioning, and neuropsychological functioning within the first hour after ECT, with fewer hemodynamic changes [43–45]. A systemic review of the effects of anesthetic agents on emergence and recovery times showed that induction agents associated with longer seizures generally have longer emergence and recovery times after ECT [44]. The mean emergence time (from drug administration to eye opening or following commands) was shorter with propofol compared to methohexital (weighted mean difference (WMD), 0.91 min) using data combined from seven crossover trials and one parallel trial and compared to thiopental (WMD, 1.75 min) using data from three crossover trials. Propofol also offers faster recovery (from initiation of general anesthesia to discharge from the PACU) compared to methohexital (WMD, 1.93 min) and thiopental (WMD, 3.40 min) using data from five crossover trials. However, if there is a need to prolong seizure duration for a successful treatment before rapid emergence or recovery, the choice of anesthetic agent should be based on the influence of each agent on seizure time, since variations in emergence and recovery times are small (although significantly different) among anesthetic agents [44].

6.2 Recovery Period

6.2.1 Postprocedural Care in the Postanesthesia Care Unit

The ECT procedure is brief and patients generally require about 2 h of post-ECT care in the PACU. An evaluation of recovery profiles after general anesthesia for acute or continuation/maintenance ambulatory ECT in a day surgery unit (DSU) [5] showed that the mean times from PACU admission until fluid intake, gait, and discharge from hospital were 55, 70, and 110 min, respectively, and that the mean total DSU stay (time to discharge from arrival at the DSU) was 172 min (Table 6.1). PACU nurses observe the patient for respiratory and cardiovascular functions, further seizure activity, and recurrent postictal agitation [46]. Some patients are hyperactive or restless, and extra nursing care or medication may be required to avoid injury to the patient or caregiver. Patients are laid on the bed with the side rail in the upright position to prevent a fall from the bed. Monitoring of SpO_2 is continued until a patient is alert, and oxygen should be given when SpO_2 falls to <90 %. Suction of the airway should be performed as needed. Noninvasive blood pressure is monitored every 5 min until the patient awakes and then every 15 min until the patient is alert. ECG monitoring should be performed when the patient is at high risk of cardiovascular disease or has a history of persistent cardiovascular events during ECT.

When vital signs are stable and the patient is alert, drinking of fluids and ambulation are permitted, as requested by the patient. PACU nurses should be vigilant regarding falls, especially for elderly patients. Patients are advised about voiding after initial ambulation. General somatic complaints (e.g., headache, muscle pain, nausea) are minor but frequent side effects after ECT as described in Section 6.2.2. These symptoms should be treated in the PACU to ensure patient comfort and enhance treatment compliance. In patients who routinely have these post-ECT complaints, administration of analgesics or antiemetics may be considered prophylactically before or at the time of future ECT.

6.2.2 Adverse Symptoms After Awareness

6.2.2.1 Headache

Post-ECT headache is a common and troubling side effect of ECT that occurs often in the initial treatment of an ECT series and particularly in young patients [1, 47]. The exact etiology is unclear, but has been postulated to involve superficial vasodilation associated with direct effects of the electrical stimulus, electrically induced contraction of temporalis and masseter muscles, or an acute increase in blood pressure [1, 47, 48]. The reported incidences of post-ECT headaches are 19, 37, and 60 % in patients receiving ECT [5, 49, 50] (Table 6.2). ECT both induces headache in previously unaffected patients and exacerbates the problem in patients with preexisting headache symptoms. Relief of post-ECT headache in most cases can be achieved with acetaminophen or nonsteroidal anti-inflammatory drugs (NSAIDs) such as ibuprofen and ketorolac. However, some patients may suffer severe headaches for several hours to several days, despite pharmacological therapy. Resistant headaches should be treated with narcotics or other medications, although narcotics may cause nausea or drowsiness and may delay recovery.

In patients who routinely have post-ECT headaches, prophylactic analgesics may be given orally before ECT or intravenously at the time of ECT. A significant subset of patients is generally ambivalent about ECT, and thus effective and

Table 6.2 Post-ECT telephone interview 24 h after ambulatory ECT (762 ambulatory ECT procedures in 40 patients) (Revised from Ref. [5])

Adverse events	Headache	144 (19 %, 23 patients)
	Muscle pain	53 (7 %, 18 patients)
	Nausea	14 (2 %, 9 patients)
	Vomiting	2 (0.3 %, 2 patients)
Medication	Analgesic agent	33 (4 %, 14 patients)
	Antiemetic agent	1 (0.1 %, 1 patient)
RNA[a]		10 (8–10)
Satisfaction[b]		10 (10–10)
Unplanned revisit to the hospital		2 (0.3 %, 2 patients[c])

Values are the number of ECT procedures (%, patient number) or median (25th–75th percentile)
RNA resumption of normal activity
[a]Resumption of normal activity: score 0 = no activity, 10 = back to normal activity
[b]Global satisfaction with ECT and anesthesia procedure: score 0 = very dissatisfied, 10 = very satisfied
[c]Both patients visited a psychiatrist due to worsening of mental status
Note: Patients characteristics are the same as those in Table 6.1

proactive analgesic therapy may promote compliance with ECT. Oral ibuprofen (600 mg) premedication 90 min before ECT was found to reduce the frequency and severity of post-ECT headache in a randomized, double-blind study, with mean visual analogue scale headache scores (0–5) that were 1.49 and 0.54 in the placebo and ibuprofen groups, respectively [50]. An antimigraine medication, sumatriptan, a serotonin subtype 5-$HT_{1B/1D}$ receptor agonist, may also be beneficial for severe vascular-like post-ECT headache [48, 51]. In an open, unblinded study in eight patients with moderate-to-severe post-ECT headaches, use of intranasal sumatriptan (20 mg) within 30 min of the initial headache complaint after ECT was found to reduce it over the subsequent 2 h [48]. In 13 patients with a history of severe post-ECT headache requiring opioid-containing analgesics, White et al. found that eight had a complete response and two had a partial response to pretreatment with intranasal sumatriptan (5 mg) 5–10 min prior to their ECT [51]. Mirtazapine is an antidepressant that antagonizes postsynaptic serotonin 5-HT_2 and 5-HT_3 receptors, and concomitant nightly administration of mirtazapine during an ECT course relieved post-ECT headache and nausea in four cases [47]. A nonpharmacologic method using a cold pack around the head after ECT in the recovery room for maximum 40 min, together with medication, has been reported to be effective for refractory headaches caused by ECT [52].

6.2.2.2 Muscle pain

Generalized muscle pain is usually caused by fasciculations associated with the depolarizing action of succinylcholine, which is routinely used in ECT as a muscle relaxant, especially in young patients. Incidence of post-ECT muscle pain has been reported 7 % (Table 6.2). Muscle pain is usually tolerable with treatment with analgesics such as acetaminophen or NSAIDs. Preemptive use of analgesics is recommended to manage refractory muscle pain. Premedication with nonparalytic doses of a nondepolarizing muscle relaxant several minutes before administration of succinylcholine is another option to prevent severe symptoms [6]. However, these muscle relaxants are competitive with succinylcholine, and thus, the dose of succinylcholine needs to be increased by 10–25 % to achieve the same degree of muscle relaxation.

6.2.2.3 Nausea

ECT-associated nausea may occur secondary to headaches or narcotics used for the treatment of headache or muscle pain or may occur independently as an adverse effect of anesthesia. The mechanism underlying ECT-associated nausea is unknown. Incidences of post-ECT nausea of 2 % and 6 % have been reported, and this complication after ECT is less frequent than headache or muscle pain [5, 20, 53] (Table 6.2). Antiemetic medication such as a dopaminergic antagonist (e.g., metoclopramide, droperidol) or 5-HT_3 receptor antagonist (e.g., ondansetron) is the most common and effective treatment for nausea. Transcutaneous acupoint electrical stimulation prior to and during ECT is an effective nonpharmacologic method for prevention of nausea in patients who have had nausea in prior ECT [53]. Post-ECT nausea may be reduced with use of propofol as an anesthetic agent. In a retrospective chart review, 7 of 340 patients treated with ECT were switched to propofol from methohexital anesthesia because of post-ECT nausea and vomiting, and these side effects were significantly reduced after this anesthetic agent change [20].

6.2.2.4 Fall

Depressed geriatric patients with unacceptable side effects from or a poor response to psychiatric medications or who have physical disorders contraindicating medications have recently become candidates for ECT. Compared with other treatment options, ECT is generally safe and effective in acute treatment of depressed elderly patients [54, 55]. However, fall is a frequent post-ECT complication, especially in geriatric patients. In an evaluation of ECT in the elderly, Cattan et al. found fall rates of 14 % in the young-old group (age 65–80 years) and 36 % in the old-old group (>80 years) [54]. A large number of ECT and Parkinson's disease are associated with higher rates of fall in the elderly population [56]. The cause of fall is multifactorial and it is difficult to determine how ECT contributes to the incidence. However, efforts at minimizing post-ECT confusion and postictal agitation may decrease the effect of ECT on fall. Elderly patients should be monitored closely after ECT not only until vital signs and consciousness return to baseline but until stable ambulation is achieved. Also, the decision to transfer from inpatient to outpatient ECT should include an assessment of the risk of fall to ensure patient safety at home [57].

6.2.3 Discharge Criteria and Patient Education in Ambulatory ECT

Discharge of patients from the PACU requires adherence to validated criteria to ensure patient safety, especially in ambulatory ECT. Each facility should have specific discharge criteria for ambulatory ECT. The criteria for discharge after ambulatory ECT include return to orientation, full alertness, stable vital signs, stable gait, and drinking of fluid [58]. Figure 6.2 shows the flow of peri-ECT anesthesia management in ambulatory ECT. Since care in ambulatory ECT is similar to care in ambulatory surgery, ambulatory ECT can be performed successfully in an ambulatory surgical center and its system [5, 46], and discharge criteria for ambulatory surgery can also be applied to ambulatory ECT. The postanesthesia discharge scoring system (PADSS) is a simple method that is widely used for uniform assessment of ambulatory surgeries and can also be applied in ambulatory ECT [5, 59]. The PADSS is a cumulative index that measures the patient's home readiness based upon five criteria: (1) vital signs, (2) ambulation, (3) pain, (4) nausea and vomiting, and (5) surgical bleeding, with each criterion scored as 0, 1, or 2. Patients with a score of 9 or higher are considered fit for discharge with a responsible adult escort. Before discharge following ambulatory ECT, a psychiatrist should assess the psychiatric status of the patient. When difficulty with patient care is expected at home based on possible changes of mental status, hospitalization should be recommended. Patients are asked about headache, muscle pain, and nausea and provided with appropriate medications. Remaining in the facility until

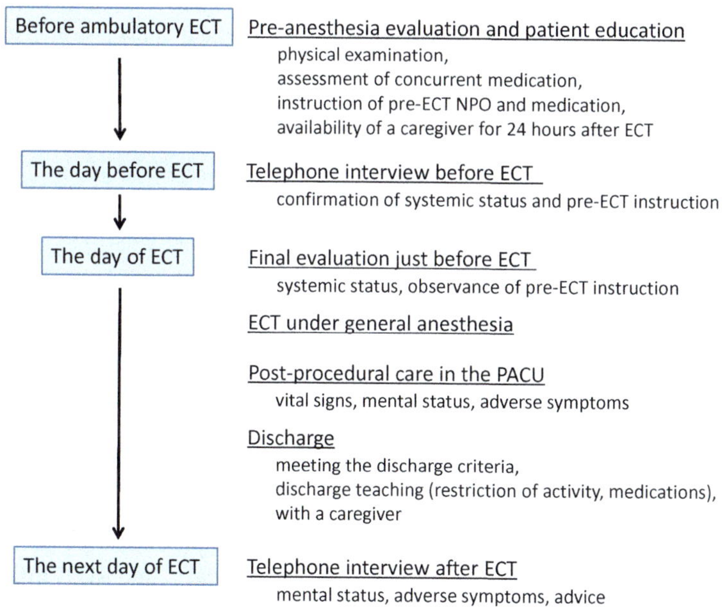

Fig. 6.2 Flow of peri-ECT anesthesia management in ambulatory ECT. *NPO* nothing per os, *PACU* postanesthesia care unit

intake of a light meal or snack and documentation of urinary output will encourage fuller recovery. For a patient requiring medications such as analgesics, sedatives, or antihypertensive drugs that prolong the recovery process in the PACU, the caregiver should be prepared for a prolonged wait after treatment.

Ambulatory ECT places more responsibility on the patient and caregiver (the family in most cases). Therefore, patient and family education is critical to the provision of safe and effective ambulatory ECT. A responsible caregiver must be available to help the patient maintain NPO status before treatment, monitor pre- and post-ECT medication, transport the patient to and from the treatment setting, stay with the patient for at least 24 h after each treatment, and provide postprocedural care at home. Patient should not return to an empty house because they have an increased risk of confusion, memory impairment, or falls at home. Patients and caregivers should be advised on concurrent and rescue medications that may be administered for postprocedural symptoms and whom to call for advice on postprocedural management. All surgical patients who received general anesthesia are instructed to avoid driving, operating machinery, or making major decisions for at least 24 h after surgery [59]. Instructions on avoiding these activities are more important for patients who have undergone ambulatory ECT, because they have a risk of cognitive impairment [46, 57]. Driving should be avoided for at least 1 week after finishing an acute ECT course (i.e., three treatments per week). If the frequency of ECT is tapered to a continuous or maintenance level, the patient should not resume driving until the frequency is once a week or less. Patients should not drive for 24 h after treatment, even if they are receiving only occasional maintenance ECT. If a patient shows any ECT-associated cognitive impairment, further restriction of driving is recommended. A psychiatrist and anesthesiologist should provide oral and written ambulatory instructions on daily living restrictions, complications and methods of treatment, the patient's medication regimen, and the 24-h emergency telephone number of the hospital.

6.3 After the Day of Treatment and Between Treatments

6.3.1 Cognitive Impairment

6.3.1.1 Memory disturbance

Anterograde and retrograde amnesia

Cognitive side effects may accumulate over repeated ECT sessions or persist beyond the course of ECT. Memory disturbance is an important cognitive impairment during and after an ECT course and may impair optimal functioning in daily living at hospital or at home. This condition comprises anterograde amnesia (difficulty in learning new information) and retrograde amnesia (difficulty in recalling information learned before ECT). Anterograde amnesia is usually restricted to the period immediately following ECT, with impairment of anterograde memory, processing speed, and working memory associated with ECT found to be mainly limited to the first 3 days posttreatment and improve after 15 days in a meta-analysis [60]. In contrast, retrograde amnesia may be more significant and require a longer period to resolve than anterograde amnesia. Post-ECT retrograde amnesia is mainly due to a temporary inability to access memories, and not to ECT permanently erasing memories. This condition generally improves over a period of weeks or months after completion of an ECT course. However, retrograde amnesia may not always completely resolve, especially for recall of the period covering the ECT. Less commonly, memory from more remote periods may be affected after a large number of bilateral ECT [1].

In a review of 10 prospective studies using brief or ultrabrief pulse unilateral ECT, Verwijk et al. assessed the severity and persistence of neurocognitive side effects of ECT such as autobiographical and anterograde verbal and nonverbal memory at 1 to 7 days (immediate), 1 to 6 months (mid-long-term) and after 6 months (long-term) post-ECT [61]. Autobiographical memory was the only cognitive function that was still impaired in the mid-long-term after ECT compared to pretreatment, but improved in this period. Anterograde verbal and nonverbal memory impairment normalized or even improved in the mid-long-term. Ultrabrief pulse ECT also caused less decline in autobiographical and anterograde memory than brief pulse ECT. In a comparison of depressed patients undergoing brief pulse bilateral ECT with matched controls, using assessment of remote memory of news over 1 year, Meeter et al. found that retrograde amnesia present within 3 days after ECT was no longer evident at 3-month follow-up, with remote memory returning to the pre-ECT level and similar to that in controls [62]. Major depression is associated with a range of cognitive deficits [63], and ECT for depression might partly be expected to improve cognitive ability concurrently with affecting the mental state.

Factors involved in cognitive impairment

Factors that may affect the extent of cognitive impairment after ECT are shown in Table 6.3. The degree and duration of cognitive change varies widely among

Table 6.3 Factors that may increase cognitive impairment after ECT

Factor	Effect
ECT parameters	
Stimulus waveform	Sine wave > brief pulse > ultrabrief pulse
Stimulus intensity	High > low
Electrode placement	Bilateral > unilateral
Number of treatments	Many > few
Frequency of treatments	Frequent > infrequent
ECT course	Index ECT > continuation/maintenance ECT
Patient parameters	
Age	Older > younger
Preexisting cognitive deficiencies	Present > absent
Educational level	Low > high

individuals and is influenced by treatment parameters such as stimulus waveform, stimulus intensity, electrode placement, frequency and number of treatments, and an index or continuation/maintenance course of ECT [1, 64]. If patients suffer from cognitive side effects during the ECT course, modification of technical factors can significantly diminish the severity of persistent ECT-related amnesia. These changes include switching from bilateral to unilateral nondominant stimulus electrode placement, switching from a brief pulse to an ultrabrief pulse stimulus, decreasing stimulus intensity, decreasing the frequency of ECT, and ensuring that the number of ECT in the index course is not greater than that required to produce a therapeutic plateau. In patients taking combinations of antidepressants, mood stabilizers, and lithium, which may themselves have a negative effect on cognitive function, discontinuing or decreasing the dosage of medications should be considered [64].

Several studies have examined the outcomes of different anesthetic agents on cognitive side effects and efficacy beyond the ECT course, as opposed to the immediate posttreatment period. Geretsegger et al. compared the effects of propofol with those of methohexital on cognitive performance in a double-blind noncrossover study of 50 ECT patients [65] and found a tendency for improved cognitive performance 8 weeks after anesthesia with propofol compared with methohexital, but with significance in only two of six cognitive trials. Vaidya et al. reviewed the records of 48 patients who received a total of 155 courses of ECT and performed a within-subject comparison of methohexital and propofol on cognitive outcome before the ECT course and within 24–48 h after ECT [66]. Mean Mini-Mental State Examination (MMSE) scores before and after ECT were similar for methohexital and propofol anesthesia. In a randomized blinded trial in 62 patients comparing propofol with thiopental, MMSE scores were 2 points lower in the propofol group 5 days after the last ECT; however, the higher number of elderly patients in the propofol group may have influenced the MMSE scores [67]. In another comparison of propofol with thiopental, Ingram et al. found slightly better anterograde verbal and visual memory 1 to 3 days after the last treatment with thiopental, but no differences 1 month later; however, the older age of the propofol group and the use of three different forms of ECT in the same group may also have confounded these results [68]. Thus, there is no clear indication of worsened cognitive function after a course of ECT with the use of methohexital, propofol, or thiopental. Use of ketamine anesthesia in ECT may be advantageous in terms of neurocognitive outcomes because of the antidepressant effect of this drug [43], and further studies measuring cognitive outcomes after an ECT course are needed to evaluate the efficacy of ketamine.

Monitoring of Cognitive Function

Routine cognitive function testing is needed before, during, and after a course of ECT [19, 64]. For example, The American Psychiatric Association Task Force Report on ECT recommends that the impact of ECT on cognitive function be assessed at least weekly and should include both objective findings and a patient report [19]. Clinicians should routinely ask patients about memory loss, and some

Table 6.4 Suggested test battery to monitor cognitive effects of ECT

Test	Domain tested	Length of test (min)	Timing of test
3MSE or MMSE	Global cognitive	10	Baseline
Hopkins verbal learning test	New learning	20	3 treatments
Autobiographical memory questionnaire – short form	Retrograde amnesia	20	6 treatments
Digit-symbol substitution task	Psychomotor speed	5	3 months post-course
Reorientation	Postictal confusion	–	After each treatment

Revised from Ref. [64]
3MSE modified mini-mental state examination, *MMSE* mini-mental state examination

conduct a personal or nonpersonal informal memory interview or simple cognitive tests such as the MMSE, which takes 5–10 min to administer and is widely understood by clinicians and frequently used for monitoring global cognitive side effects associated with ECT [60]. The MMSE is sufficiently sensitive to detect differences in cognitive side effects in follow-up of patients 6 months after treatment at different hospitals using different ECT techniques [69]. Porter et al. suggested a test battery and suitable timing to monitor cognitive effects of ECT (Table 6.4) [64], in which detailed cognitive tests are carried out at baseline, after three and six treatments of ECT, and at 2 to 3 months after the ECT course using the same battery. The approximate time to reorientation should be measured after each treatment. Detailed monitoring of cognitive function during the course of ECT allows detection of cognitive changes at an earlier stage and better planning of future treatment such as electrode placement, dose of electricity, frequency of treatments, and timing of treatment termination. However, a neuropsychological battery lasting 2–3 h is unlikely to be tolerated or to be practical for routine clinical use, especially for severely depressed patients. Since patients' complaints of memory dysfunction following ECT are related more to self-perception than to scores on a test battery, asking patients about memory impairment should always be a part of assessment of the effects of ECT [1].

6.3.1.2 Confusion

Postictal confusion generally disappears over a period of days after an ECT course, but occasionally may not fully disappear and may progress to an interictal confusion state. The sudden onset of this state, particularly within hours or days after an ECT session, is a cause for concern and must be quickly assessed. A variety of factors may be involved, including a recent medication change, substance abuse or withdrawal, acute exposure to toxic substances, nonconvulsive status epilepticus, or an acute dissociative state [1]. If nonconvulsive status epilepticus is considered as an emergency, an EEG should be obtained. If severe postictal confusion occurs at home, the caregiver should report this to an attending psychiatrist or the ECT team.

6.3.2 Postprocedural Care at Home

There has been a recent shift from inpatient to ambulatory ECT, since ambulatory ECT minimizes the cost of hospitalization and allows patients to receive treatment with less disruption to normal routines. However, a disadvantage of ambulatory ECT is the reduced opportunity to monitor the treatment response and adverse effects, in comparison with inpatient treatment [70]. Ambulatory ECT is as safe and effective as inpatient ECT in medically and socially screened patients and is accepted by most patients [5, 71, 72]; however, follow-up after treatment is an important part of perioperative management of ambulatory ECT to assess mental status, identify adverse events, give advice to patients and caregivers, increase their satisfaction, and improve the practice. Typically, telephone assessments of mood and adverse effects are conducted the day after each ambulatory ECT (Fig. 6.2) [5, 57, 58]. Headache and muscle pain are the two most common systemic side effects in telephone coverage on the day after ambulatory ECT (Table 6.2). Advice on medication and care for each symptom are given to patients or caregivers. Rather than such symptoms, deterioration of mental status or confusion can be a cause of an unplanned revisit to the hospital [5], and a few depressed patients with bipolar disorders can become manic during the course of ECT. If memory disturbance, confusion, or deterioration of mental status emerge following ECT, caregivers should help the patient manage activities of daily living by carefully monitoring the medication regimen, maintaining a driving restriction, and being vigilant with regard to the increased risk of falls [57]. Home nursing can avoid ECT-associated cognitive impairment leading to inpatient hospitalization. If the patient has a psychiatric condition or significant cognitive impairment that results in failure of home nursing, emergency readmission may be warranted. Daily monitoring of the ambulatory ECT response and adverse effects through an interactive voice system that allows patients to report symptoms via an automated telephone interview has been used to obtain detailed information that can enhance clinical decision making [70]. Thus, a 24-h emergency support system for the patient and caregivers is necessary in ambulatory ECT.

There is no fixed convalescent period for ambulatory ECT. Cognitive impairment after the course of ECT is one notable difference in postoperative care between patients who undergo ambulatory surgery and those who receive ambulatory ECT. When, and to what degree, patients may assume responsible work or return to school, use complex mechanical equipment, or make financial decisions should be discussed with the patient and caregivers repeatedly over the course of ECT, based on the severity of the patient's disorder, cognitive performance, physical status, and the requirements of the patient's work [57, 58]. Adding to the interval after ECT, concurrent psychotropic medications that might be sedating should be considered in making a decision about driving (see

Section 6.2.3). The treating psychiatrist is responsible for clinical care at home throughout the course of ambulatory ECT, by assessment of progression of symptoms, adverse events, signs of relapse, and concurrent medication.

6.3.3 Programmatic Considerations

6.3.3.1 Index ECT and Continuation/Maintenance ECT

Most ECT are administered two or three times a week in the index (acute) course, typically with total 6–12 treatments for relief of acute symptoms, although as many as 20 are occasionally required. Treatment frequency may be increased to daily if a more rapid response is needed, particularly early in the course. Decreasing the treatment frequency to twice or even once weekly should be considered if cognitive side effects are severe. When a patient is judged to have shown a maximum clinical response, the ECT course is terminated. Two or three additional treatments are needed to show a plateau in improvement. Alterations in the ECT course, ECT and anesthetic parameters, should be considered for nonresponders or patients whose clinical progress is minimal after approximately 6 treatments. Possible modifications include changing the electrode placement, stimulus intensity, anesthetic agent and dose, or potentiating the seizure pharmacologically. If the patient does not respond after 3–4 additional treatments, the ECT course should be terminated.

After a successful index course of ECT, prevention of relapse and prolonged remission are important issues. Relapse rates exceed 50 % after successful treatment with ECT, and relapse tends to occur within the first 6 months after the immediate phase [73]. After successful treatment with ECT, patients require pharmacotherapy, continuation/maintenance ECT, or both to reduce this risk. Continuation/maintenance ECT is an effective and safe treatment option for relapse prevention, even in elderly patients [73–75]. In general, continuation ECT is defined as treatment within 6 months to prevent relapse after remission due to the index course of ECT. Maintenance ECT is administered after this 6-month period and indicated for patients with recurrent and treatment-resistance conditions. Criteria for continuation ECT include all of the following: a history of recurrent illness that is acutely responsive to ECT; limited medical comorbidities that increase the risk for additional ECT or anesthesia; ineffectiveness or intolerance to prophylaxis with pharmacotherapy or patient preference for additional ECT; and ability and willingness to comply with logistical arrangements because continuation ECT is often performed on an outpatient basis [74]. Typically, continuation ECT begins with one ECT weekly, gradually extending to once every other week, once every month, and once every other month. When patients have frequent relapse or recurrence of illness, an increase in frequency of treatments, extension of the treatment period, or a restart of index ECT may be considered. The appearance of recurring symptoms, as demonstrated in a mental status examination or reported by a patient or caregiver, provides clues to the optimal treatment schedule. Continuation/maintenance ECT does not have a fixed end point, and termination is determined empirically. This form of ECT should be administered at the minimum frequency and numbers to prevent relapse. Some patients require treatment over years due to the severity and chronicity of their condition, especially when attempts to discontinue therapy result in recurrence. Determination and documentation of the continued need for ECT should be made periodically based on assessment of the relevant benefits and risks, and informed consent should be obtained from the patient and family at least every 6 months [74].

6.3.3.2 Inpatient and Ambulatory ECT

Index courses of ECT are combined in inpatient and ambulatory care settings. As a general rule, it is advisable for patients who have never or not recently had ECT to have a brief inpatient admission to receive ECT, during which their response to the treatment can be closely observed [57]. Such admission is always advisable for patients with unstable medical complications, especially cardiac or respiratory complications; potential medical complications that could arise from the treatment; adverse behaviors such as suicide, harm to others, and excitement; and significant anxiety or ambivalence about receiving ECT. A patient who resides too far from the facility is not a good candidate for ambulatory ECT. If the patient does not meet the above criteria and is able to maintain adequate self-care (activities of daily living, medications) and NPO status before ECT, and a support person is available to supervise the patient (see Section 6.2.3), ambulatory ECT is safely initiated, even in the index course of ECT.

In making the decision to switch from inpatient to ambulatory ECT, the following issues should be considered during hospitalization [57]: (1) How well the patient recovers from each treatment, including reorientation, drowsiness in the afternoon posttreatment, and the severity of ECT side effects (e.g., lingering headache, nausea or muscle pain), since these factors will affect safety at home. (2) Cognitive status, especially memory impairment, taking into account the level of support the patient will receive at home. A safety evaluation by an occupational therapist may be helpful. (3) Assessment of the posttreatment risk for fall made by inpatient staff, especially in patients who are elderly or have unstable gait or blood pressure.

If the patient tolerates and responds well to the treatment in the index course of ECT as an inpatient, he or she can be discharged after several treatments and receive further ECT as an outpatient. If treatments are medically or socially complicated, the index course of ECT needs to be completed as an inpatient. Safe ambulatory ECT requires cooperation of the patient and family, and the patient should complete a new informed consent process for ambulatory ECT in the presence of their family when transitioning from inpatient ECT.

Continuation/maintenance ECT is well tolerated and often performed as ambulatory ECT. Patients who need continuation/maintenance ECT after a successful index course generally have a predictable response to ECT and a stable mental status. The lower frequency of continuation/maintenance ECT also results in fewer cognitive side effects compared to those in the index course, which contributes to safety at home. Ambulatory ECT also offers more flexible scheduling of ECT linked to treatment response, regardless of space in the ward, and can minimize or preclude the appearance of recurrent symptoms. These advantages result in a high completion rate of scheduled ECT and low dropout rate for ambulatory continuation/maintenance ECT [71, 72].

Close integration of inpatient and ambulatory ECT is crucial for safety and to ensure a seamless transition in either direction [19]. If the patient cannot continue ambulatory ECT because of a change of medical status or home environment, a transition to inpatient ECT is necessary. Medical record keeping for ambulatory ECT follows the same standard as that for inpatient ECT. Before ECT, regardless of inpatient or outpatient, the treatment team (psychiatrists, anesthesiologists, and nurses) should assess the method of ECT management, adverse effects from earlier ECT, and ongoing medical conditions that may affect the risks or benefits of future ECT.

In ambulatory ECT, systemic reexaminations and laboratory tests vary with the physical status of the patient during the ECT course and with institutional policy. For patients in good health with no new signs of systemic disorder, these are usually updated semiannually or at least yearly [58]. For patients under treatment for systemic disorders (e.g., diabetes, hypertension, asthma), medical review and laboratory tests are periodically repeated every few weeks to every 6 months, based on individual needs and medical conditions. If signs of systemic disorder worsen or new signs emerge between treatments, a medical review and laboratory tests or consultation with a specialist are required prior to the next treatment.

References

1. Mankad MV, Weiner RD. Adverse effects. In: Mankad MV, Beyer JL, Weiner RD, Krystal AD, editors. Clinical manual of electroconvulsive therapy. Arlington: American Psychiatric Publishing, Inc.; 2010. p. 139–48.
2. Auriacombe M, Rénéric JP, Usandizaga D, Gomez F, Combourieu I, Tignol J. Post-ECT agitation and plasma lactate concentrations. J ECT. 2000;16:263–7.
3. Cristancho MA, Alici Y, Augoustides JG, O'Reardon JP. Uncommon but serious complications associated with electroconvulsive therapy: recognition and management for the clinician. Curr Psychiatry Rep. 2008;10:474–80.
4. Kikuchi A, Yasui-Furukori N, Fujii A, Katagai H, Kaneko S. Identification of predictors of post-ictal delirium after electroconvulsive therapy. Psychiatry Clin Neurosci. 2009;63:180–5.
5. Sato M, Hirota K, Shirakami G, Kakuyama M, Tanabe H, Fukuda K. Safety in general anesthesia for ambulatory electroconvulsive therapy. Masui. 2013;62:52–9.
6. Mankad MV, Weiner RD. Anesthetics and other medications. In: Mankad MV, Beyer JL, Weiner RD, Krystal AD, editors. Clinical manual of electroconvulsive therapy. Arlington: American Psychiatric Publishing, Inc.; 2010. p. 81–93.
7. Augoustides JG, Greenblatt E, Abbas MA, O'Reardon JP, Datto CJ. Clinical approach to agitation after electroconvulsive therapy: a case report and literature review. J ECT. 2002;18:213–7.
8. O'Reardon JP, Takieddine N, Datto CJ, Augoustides JG. Propofol for the management of emergence agitation after electroconvulsive therapy: review of a case series. J ECT. 2006;22:247–52.

9. Tzabazis A, Schmitt HJ, Ihmsen H, Schmidtlein M, Zimmermann R, Wielopolski J, et al. Postictal agitation after electroconvulsive therapy: incidence, severity, and propofol as a treatment option. J ECT. 2013;29:189–95.
10. Mizrak A, Koruk S, Ganidagli S, Bulut M, Oner U. Premedication with dexmedetomidine and midazolam attenuates agitation after electroconvulsive therapy. J Anesth. 2009;23:6–10.
11. O'Brien EM, Rosenquist PB, Kimball JN, Dunn GN, Smith B, Arias LM. Dexmedetomidine and the successful management of electroconvulsive therapy postictal agitation: a case report. J ECT. 2010;26:131–3.
12. Bryson EO, Briggs MC, Pasculli RM, Kellner CH. Treatment-resistant postictal agitation after electroconvulsive therapy (ECT) controlled with dexmedetomidine. J ECT. 2013;29, e18.
13. Vishne T, Amiaz R, Grunhaus L. Promethazine for the treatment of agitation after electroconvulsive therapy: a case series. J ECT. 2005;21:118–21.
14. Small JG, Milstein V. Lithium interactions: lithium and electroconvulsive therapy. J Clin Psychopharmacol. 1990;10:346–50.
15. Prudic J. Strategies to minimize cognitive side effects with ECT: aspects of ECT technique. J ECT. 2008;24:46–51.
16. Swartz CM. Electroconvulsive therapy emergence agitation and succinylcholine dose. J Nerv Ment Dis. 1990;178:455–7.
17. Devanand DP, Sackeim HA. Use of increased anesthetic dose prior to electroconvulsive therapy to prevent postictal excitement. Gen Hosp Psychiatry. 1992;14:345–9.
18. Reti IM, Krishnan A, Podlisky A, Sharp A, Walker M, Neufeld KJ, et al. Predictors of electroconvulsive therapy postictal delirium. Psychosomatics. 2014;55:272–9.
19. American Psychiatric Association Committee on Electroconvulsive Therapy. The practice of electroconvulsive therapy: Recommendations for treatment, training, and privileging. 2nd ed. Washington, DC: American Psychiatric Association; 2001.
20. Bailine SH, Petrides G, Doft M, Lui G. Indications for the use of propofol in electroconvulsive therapy. J ECT. 2003;19:129–32.
21. Krystal AD. Managing the ECT seizure. In: Mankad MV, Beyer JL, Weiner RD, Krystal AD, editors. Clinical manual of electroconvulsive therapy. Arlington: American Psychiatric Publishing, Inc.; 2010. p. 149–57.
22. Avramov MN, Husain MM, White PF. The comparative effects of methohexital, propofol, and etomidate for electroconvulsive therapy. Anesth Analg. 1995;81:596–602.
23. Lowenstein DH, Alldredge BK. Status epilepticus. N Engl J Med. 1998;338:970–6.
24. Saito S. Anesthesia management for electroconvulsive therapy: hemodynamic and respiratory management. J Anesth. 2005;19:142–9.
25. Saito S, Kadoi Y, Nihishara F, Aso C, Goto F. End-tidal carbon dioxide monitoring stabilized hemodynamic changes during ECT. J ECT. 2003;19:26–30.
26. Mayur PM, Shree RS, Gangadhar BN, Subbakrishna DK, Janakiramaiah N, Rao GS. Atropine premedication and the cardiovascular response to electroconvulsive therapy. Br J Anaesth. 1998;81:466–7.
27. Ding Z, White PF. Anesthesia for electroconvulsive therapy. Anesth Analg. 2002;94:1351–64.
28. Tecoult E, Nathan N. Morbidity in electroconvulsive therapy. Eur J Anaesthesiol. 2001;18:511–8.
29. McCormick AS, Saunders DA. Oxygen saturation of patients recovering from electroconvulsive therapy. Anaesthesia. 1996;51:702–4.
30. Wayne SL, O'Donovan CA, McCall WV, Link K. Postictal neurogenic pulmonary edema: experience from an ECT model. Convuls Ther. 1997;13:181–4.
31. Kurnutala LN, Kamath S, Koyfman S, Yarmush J, SchianodiCola J. Aspiration during electroconvulsive therapy under general anesthesia. J ECT. 2013;29, e68.
32. Burke WJ, Rubin EH, Zorumski CF, Wetzel RD. The safety of ECT in geriatric psychiatry. J Am Geriatr Soc. 1987;35:516–21.
33. Buisseret P. Acute pulmonary edema following grand mal epilepsy and as a complication of electric shock therapy. Br J Dis Chest. 1982;76:194–5.

34. Takahashi T, Kinoshita K, Fuke T, Urushihata K, Kawamata T, Yanagisawa S, et al. Acute neurogenic pulmonary edema following electroconvulsive therapy: a case report. Gen Hosp Psychiatry. 2012;34:703.e9–703.e11.
35. Myers CL, Gopalka A, Glick D, Goldman MB, Dinwiddie SH. A case of negative-pressure pulmonary edema after electroconvulsive therapy. J ECT 2007;23:281–3.
36. Cochran M, DeBattista C, Schmiesing C, Brock-Utne JG. Negative-pressure pulmonary edema: a potential hazard in patients undergoing ECT. J ECT. 1999;15:168–70.
37. Weber DL, Ruvolo C, Cashin P. Sudden death following electroconvulsive therapy. N Y State J Med. 1973;73:1000–1.
38. Mamah D, Lammle M, Isenberg KE. Pulmonary embolism after ECT. J ECT. 2005;21:39–40.
39. Singh G, Wahi S. Pulmonary embolism in the ECT patient: a case report and discussion. Gen Hosp Psychiatry. 2008;30:87–9.
40. Mehta V, Mueller PS, Gonzalez-Arriaza HL, Pankratz VS, Rummans TA. Safety of electroconvulsive therapy in patients receiving long-term warfarin therapy. Mayo Clin Proc. 2004;79:1396–401.
41. Saito S, Kadoi Y, Iriuchijima N, Obata H, Arai K, Morita T, et al. Reduction of cerebral hyperemia with anti-hypertensive medication after electroconvulsive therapy. Can J Anaesth. 2000;47:767–74.
42. Sundsted KK, Burton MC, Shah R, Lapid MI. Preanesthesia medical evaluation for electroconvulsive therapy: a review of the literature. J ECT. 2014;30:35–42.
43. MacPherson RD, Loo CK. Cognitive impairment following electroconvulsive therapy – does the choice of anesthetic agent make a difference? J ECT. 2008;24:52–6.
44. Hooten WM, Rasmussen KG. Effects of general anesthetic agents in adults receiving electroconvulsive therapy: a systematic review. J ECT. 2008;24:208–23.
45. Rasmussen KG. Propofol for ECT anesthesia a review of the literature. J ECT. 2014;30:210–5.
46. Irvin SM. Treatment of depression with outpatient electroconvulsive therapy. AORN J. 1997;65:573–82.
47. Li TC, Shiah IS, Sun CJ, Tzang RF, Huang KC, Lee WK. Mirtazapine relieves post-electroconvulsive therapy headaches and nausea: a case series and review of the literature. J ECT. 2011;27:165–7.
48. Markowitz JS, Kellner CH, DeVane CL, Beale MD, Folk J, Burns C, et al. Intranasal sumatriptan in post-ECT headache: results of an open-label trial. J ECT. 2001;17:280–3.
49. Weiner SJ, Ward TN, Ravaris CL. Headache and electroconvulsive therapy. Headache. 1994;34:155–9.
50. Leung M, Hollander Y, Brown GR. Pretreatment with ibuprofen to prevent electroconvulsive therapy-induced headache. J Clin Psychiatry. 2003;64:551–3.
51. White PF, Purdue L, Downing M, Thornton L. Intranasal sumatriptan for prevention of post-ECT headaches. Headache. 2006;46:692.
52. Kramer BA, Kadar AG, Clark K. Use of the Neuro-Wrap system for severe post-electroconvulsive therapy headaches. J ECT. 2008;24:152–5.
53. Kramer BA, Kadar AG, Clark K. Transcutaneous acupoint electrical stimulation in preventing and treating nausea and vomiting in patients receiving electroconvulsive therapy. J ECT. 2003;19:194–6.
54. Cattan RA, Barry PP, Mead G, Reefe WE, Gay A, Silverman M. Electroconvulsive therapy in octogenarians. J Am Geriatr Soc. 1990;38:753–8.
55. van der Wurff FB, Stek ML, Hoogendijk WJ, Beekman AT. The efficacy and safety of ECT in depressed older adults: a literature review. Int J Geriatr Psychiatry. 2003;18:894–904.
56. de Carle AJ, Kohn R. Electroconvulsive therapy and falls in the elderly. J ECT. 2000;16:252–7.
57. Reti IM, Walker M, Pulia K, Gallegos J, Jayaram G, Vaidya P. Safety considerations for outpatient electroconvulsive therapy. J Psychiatr Pract. 2012;18:130–6.
58. Fink M, Abrams R, Bailine S, Jaffe R. Ambulatory electroconvulsive therapy: report of a task force of the association for convulsive therapy. Convuls Ther. 1996;12:42–55.

59. Awad IT, Chung F. Factors affecting recovery and discharge following ambulatory surgery. Can J Anaesth. 2006;53:858–72.
60. Semkovska M, McLoughlin DM. Objective cognitive performance associated with electroconvulsive therapy for depression: a systematic review and meta-analysis. Biol Psychiatry. 2010;68:568–77.
61. Verwijk E, Comijs HC, Kok RM, Spaans HP, Stek ML, Scherder EJ. Neurocognitive effects after brief pulse and ultrabrief pulse unilateral electroconvulsive therapy for major depression: a review. J Affect Disord. 2012;140:233–43.
62. Meeter M, Murre JM, Janssen SM, Birkenhager T, van den Broek WW. Retrograde amnesia after electroconvulsive therapy: a temporary effect? J Affect Disord. 2011;132:216–22.
63. Herrmann LL, Goodwin GM, Ebmeier KP. The cognitive neuropsychology of depression in the elderly. Psychol Med. 2007;37:1693–702.
64. Porter RJ, Douglas K, Knight RG. Monitoring of cognitive effects during a course of electroconvulsive therapy: recommendations for clinical practice. J ECT. 2008;24:25–34.
65. Geretsegger C, Nickel M, Judendorfer B, Rochowanski E, Novak E, Aichhorn W. Propofol and methohexital as anesthetic agents for electroconvulsive therapy: a randomized, double-blind comparison of electroconvulsive therapy seizure quality, therapeutic efficacy, and cognitive performance. J ECT. 2007;23:239–43.
66. Vaidya PV, Anderson EL, Bobb A, Pulia K, Jayaram G, Reti I. A within-subject comparison of propofol and methohexital anesthesia for electroconvulsive therapy. J ECT. 2012;28:14–9.
67. Bauer J, Hageman I, Dam H, Báez A, Bolwig T, Roed J, et al. Comparison of propofol and thiopental as anesthetic agents for electroconvulsive therapy: a randomized, blinded comparison of seizure duration, stimulus charge, clinical effect, and cognitive side effects. J ECT. 2009;25:85–90.
68. Ingram A, Schweitzer I, Ng CH, Saling MM, Savage G. A comparison of propofol and thiopentone use in electroconvulsive therapy: cognitive and efficacy effects. J ECT. 2007;23:158–62.
69. Sackeim HA, Prudic J, Fuller R, Keilp J, Lavori PW, Olfson M. The cognitive effects of electroconvulsive therapy in community settings. Neuropsychopharmacology. 2007;32:244–54.
70. Fazzino TL, Rabinowitz T, Althoff RR, Helzer JE. Monitoring daily affective symptoms and memory function using interactive voice response in outpatients receiving electroconvulsive therapy. J ECT. 2013;29:318–24.
71. Jaffe R, Dubin W, Shoyer B, Roemer R, Sharon D, Lipschutz L. Outpatient electroconvulsive therapy: efficacy and safety. Convuls Ther. 1990;6:231–8.
72. Dew R, McCall WV. Efficiency of outpatient ECT. J ECT. 2004;20:24–5.
73. Trevino K, McClintock SM, Husain MM. A review of continuation electroconvulsive therapy: application, safety, and efficacy. J ECT. 2010;26:186–95.
74. Petrides G, Tobias KG, Kellner CH, Rudorfer MV. Continuation and maintenance electroconvulsive therapy for mood disorders: review of the literature. Neuropsychobiology. 2011;64:129–40.
75. van Schaik AM, Comijs HC, Sonnenberg CM, Beekman AT, Sienaert P, Stek ML. Efficacy and safety of continuation and maintenance electroconvulsive therapy in depressed elderly patients: a systematic review. Am J Geriatr Psychiatry. 2012;20:5–17.

Complication of Electroconvulsive Therapy 7

Zen'ichiro Wajima

Abstract

Electroconvulsive therapy (ECT) procedures have risks, and these risks are associated with general anesthesia, tonic-clonic seizure and convulsion, the interaction between concomitant medications and ECT, and other procedural aspects of ECT. Based on the findings of a recent paper, ECT may be safer than is widely reported. The reported adverse events were mostly rare and generally minor in severity. According to the American Psychiatric Association, ECT has no absolute contraindications; however, some conditions pose a relatively high risk, and there are many other kinds of complications associated with ECT, with the cause of death during ECT essentially being from cardiovascular disorder. Understanding such complications and their management strategies avoids unnecessary discontinuation of treatment due to manageable ECT complications, and furthermore, ECT clinicians must also consider the risk-benefit ratio when treating high-risk and medically complicated patients. Moreover, anesthesiologists must evaluate risk factors carefully prior to ECT and pay attention to modifications in patient management or ECT technique that may diminish the level of risk. To avoid complications, it is very important that the anesthesiologist perform a pre-ECT evaluation. Proper anesthetic care also allows safe administration of ECT in patients with multiple coexisting medical conditions and even in very elderly patients.

Z. Wajima (✉)
Department of Anesthesiology, International University of Health and Welfare Shioya Hospital, 77 Tomita, Yaita, Tochigi 329-2145, Japan

Department of Anesthesiology, International University of Health and Welfare Hospital, 537-3 Iguchi, Nasu-Shiobara, Tochigi 329-2763, Japan
e-mail: HFB01245@nifty.com

S. Saito (ed.), *Anesthesia Management for Electroconvulsive Therapy*,
DOI 10.1007/978-4-431-55717-3_7

Keywords
Cardiovascular complication • Respiratory complication • Central nervous system complication • Postictal agitation and delirium • Allergic reaction

7.1 Pantography

Electroconvulsive therapy (ECT) procedures have risks, and these risks are associated with general anesthesia, tonic-clonic seizure and convulsion, the interaction between concomitant medications and ECT, and other aspects of the ECT procedure [1]. The estimated overall mortality rate from ECT in a general population of patients was reported to be extremely low, 2–10 per 100,000 patients [1, 2], and the cause of death during ECT is essentially from cardiovascular disorder [3]. However, over the last 30 years, substantial improvements have been made in both anesthesiology safety and ECT technique that have resulted in lower rates of mortality [4]. For example, Shiwach et al. [5] examined the mandatory reports of all deaths that occurred within 14 days of ECT and found a rate of less than two deaths per 100,000 ECT treatments. Nuttall et al. [6] found no deaths in more than 17,000 ECT treatments performed in a single hospital between 1999 and 2003. A recent report using the Veterans Affairs National Center for Patient Safety database for reports of adverse events related to ECT showed that the mortality rate associated with ECT was less than one death per 73,440 treatments [4]. Therefore, it is possible that the widely cited rates of adverse events do not apply to ECT as currently practiced [4]. Nonetheless, there are many other kinds of complications associated with ECT. According to the American Psychiatric Association (APA) [1, 7], ECT has no absolute contraindications; however, certain conditions pose a relatively high risk: (1) unstable or severe cardiovascular conditions such as recent myocardial infarction, unstable angina, poorly compensated congestive heart failure, and severe valvular cardiac disease; (2) aneurysm or vascular malformation possibly susceptible to rupture with increased blood pressure; (3) increased intracranial pressure, as may occur with some brain tumors or other space-occupying cerebral lesions; (4) recent cerebral infarction and hemorrhage; (5) pulmonary conditions such as severe chronic obstructive pulmonary disease, asthma, or pneumonia; (6) patient status rated as American Society of Anesthesiologists (ASA) level 4 or 5; and (7) pheochromocytoma. Anesthesiologists must evaluate risk factors carefully prior to ECT and must pay attention to modifications in patient management or ECT technique that may diminish the level of risk. To avoid the complications, it is very important that the anesthesiologist perform a pre-ECT evaluation. Proper anesthetic care also allows safe administration of ECT in patients with multiple coexisting medical conditions and even in very elderly patients [8–10]. Understanding such complications and their management strategies avoids unnecessary discontinuation of treatment due to manageable ECT complications [11], and furthermore, ECT clinicians must also consider the risk-benefit ratio when treating high-risk and medically complicated patients.

7.2 Cardiovascular Complications

7.2.1 General Issues

Both the stimulus of ECT and the induced seizure cause a parasympathetic and sympathetic reaction, respectively [10]. The first reaction is mediated through stimulation of the vagus nerve and ends when the actual seizure starts, usually within seconds [10], and bradycardia or frank asystole may persist [12–15]. Premature atrial and ventricular contractions, or a combination of these arrhythmias, and hypotension also may be observed [9]. One study showed that transient decreases in left ventricular ejection fraction were detected in approximately one-third of the patients after the first treatment, although these changes were not clinically apparent [16]. Hase et al. [17] observed cardiac movement during electrical stimulation using thoracic echocardiography and found that asystole, which was defined as the absence of a heartbeat for over 2 s, was observed in 48.7 % of the patients studied. The second reaction, amplified by the release of catecholamines, may last several minutes [10], at which time the heart rate and arterial pressure increase dramatically [10, 18–21]. During a seizure, an intense sympathetic discharge is transmitted directly to the cardiovascular system via the spinal sympathetic tract, causing tachycardia, hypertension, and premature ventricular contractions, and, rarely, ventricular tachycardia [9, 14]. Tachy-/bradyarrhythmias and hypertensive crises are seen more frequently than are more serious complications such as myocardial infarction, pulmonary edema, cardiac rupture, or asystole [22–24]. These complications tend to occur especially in patients with a prior history of cardiovascular disease [22–24]. ECT has been found to be relatively safe even in high-risk cardiac patients, as long as careful management is provided [6, 9, 25]. Alpak et al. [24] recommend that ECT teams (the psychiatrists, anesthesiologists, and nurses involved) should be aware of increased sympathetic tone and observe patients for at least 20 min after each ECT session and that ECT units include a recovery room.

7.2.2 Drugs to Treat the Hyperdynamic State

The tachycardia generally peaks at 2 min after the stimulus and is normally self-limiting [26]. Severe elevations in blood pressure and heart rate during ECT may have an unfavorable effect on the myocardial oxygen supply and demand ratio and can increase the risk of myocardial infarction or stroke in susceptible patients [26]. Other patients at risk include those with brain tumors, cardiac conduction defects or ectopy, hypertension, recent myocardial infarction or hemorrhagic stroke, and aortic or cerebral aneurysms [26].

Many drugs, including nitroglycerine [27, 28]; nitroprusside [29]; α_2 agonist such as clonidine [30]; opioids such as alfentanil [31] and remifentanil [31, 32]; calcium channel blockers such as nifedipine [33–35], nicardipine [36], diltiazem [18], and verapamil [19]; β-adrenergic blockers such as esmolol [37–43] and landiolol [21]; and α- and β-adrenergic blockers such as labetalol [36, 40, 42, 44–46], attenuate the hyperdynamic responses to ECT. Pretreatment with these antihypertensives and also opioids is common in patients with impaired cardiovascular and intracerebral physiology (ASA physical status III and IV) presenting for ECT [26]. Prophylactic use of β-adrenergic blocking agents such as labetalol or esmolol has become more common with the goal of lessening the hypertensive and tachycardic effects of seizure induction [47]. Nevertheless, the routine use of a prophylactic β-blocker, especially esmolol, is controversial [48]. Several studies have shown that esmolol has no effect on the duration of seizures [37, 40], whereas other studies have shown a shortened duration of seizures in patients treated with esmolol [38, 39, 41, 43], and it remains uncertain whether the potential reduction in seizure duration leads to reduced treatment efficacy [48]. Tess and Smetana et al. [48] believe that the risk-benefit calculation favors selective rather than universal use for patients who are not already receiving a β-adrenergic blocker and who do not meet independent criteria for β-adrenergic blockade therapy. Because the potential for reduced efficacy of ECT outweighs any potential benefit of β-adrenergic blockers in low-risk patients, they recommend reserving the use of prophylactic, short-acting intravenous β-adrenergic blockers for patients at high risk for complications, such as those with previous prolonged hypertension or a coexisting condition that requires tight blood pressure control (e.g., moderate or severe aortic stenosis, intracranial or other aneurysms, or recent myocardial ischemia or infarction) [48]. Remifentanil, a potent synthetic opioid that provides a rapid onset and brief duration of general anesthesia, is associated with longer seizure durations when used as the sole anesthetic or as an adjunct when the dose of the primary anesthetic is lowered [32]. Furthermore, data on hemodynamic effects are mixed but suggest favorable effects with remifentanil when seizure duration was not prolonged [32], and therefore, the use of remifentanil may be an option in the ECT procedure.

7.2.3 Cardiac Arrhythmias

Cardiac arrhythmias are probably the most significant complications of ECT [4]. However, the arrhythmias associated with ECT, even in patients with preexisting arrhythmias, are self-limiting and are not in themselves a contraindication to treatment [9].

7.2.4 Cardiac Arrest

Cardiac arrest during ECT has been reported, although it rarely occurs in current practice [49–51], and there have also been reports of severe bradycardia [51, 52]. Transient asystole secondary to parasympathetic discharge during delivery of the stimulus is rare during ECT; however, it may be prevented with pretreatment with an anticholinergic [9]. Glycopyrrolate is preferred over atropine because it produces less tachycardia after ECT [9, 26].

7.2.5 ECG Changes

Transient ECG changes, including ST-segment depression and T-wave inversion, may also be seen after ECT without any of the myocardial enzyme changes associated with myocardial infarction [9]. These ECG changes are presumed to be secondary to the sympathetic discharge [9, 53, 54].

7.2.6 Acute Myocardial Infarction and Ischemic Changes

Acute myocardial infarction and cardiac tamponade secondary to cardiac rupture are also reported as complications of ECT, although they are uncommon [53, 55, 56]. Messina et al. [57] showed that ECT causes ischemic changes and segmental wall motion abnormalities observed on echocardiography in patients with cardiovascular disease or risk factors for atherosclerosis. Myocardial stunning refers to contractile dysfunction that persists after an ischemic episode and restoration of coronary blood flow but with eventual complete recovery; there have been several case reports of myocardial stunning following ECT [58].

7.2.7 Takotsubo Cardiomyopathy

Takotsubo cardiomyopathy is a novel acute cardiac syndrome characterized by transient regional systolic dysfunction of the left ventricular apex and mid-ventricle, with hyperkinesis of the basal left ventricular segments, that has been associated with severe emotional or physical stress, and Takotsubo cardiomyopathy has been identified as a potential complication of ECT [59–62]. There are no formal guidelines in place for the treatment of Takotsubo cardiomyopathy, especially in the setting of ECT [61]. In the acute setting of Takotsubo cardiomyopathy, owing to its similarities with acute coronary syndrome, patients typically are treated with a combination of β-adrenergic blockers, aspirin, nitrates, and heparin; vasopressors may be added if cardiac function is severely impaired [61]. For maintenance treatment, patients are often maintained on a combination of angiotensin-converting enzyme inhibitors, angiotensin receptor blockers, β-adrenergic blockers, calcium channel blockers, and/or aspirin [61, 63].

7.2.8 Arrhythmias in Patients with Cardiac Rhythm Management Devices and Implantable Cardioverter-Defibrillators

ECT in patients with cardiac rhythm management devices may induce premature ventricular contractions, supraventricular tachycardia, and asystole [64], and these patients require particular attention because no controlled trials exist to support current empirical recommendations [64]. Meanwhile, Gosselink et al. commented that studies have shown that the risks of pacemaker malfunction or cardiac complications during ECT are relatively small [65]. Dolenc et al. [66] reviewed their experience in treating 26 pacemaker patients and three implantable cardioverter-defibrillator (ICD) patients with ECT. Only one serious cardiac event occurred, that of supraventricular tachycardia requiring a stay on the cardiac intensive care unit. They concluded from this experience that with proper pre-ECT cardiac and pacemaker/defibrillator assessment, ECT can be safely and effectively administered to patients with an implanted cardiac device [66]. The recommendations for patients with an implanted pacemaker are to test the pacemaker before and after ECT and to place a magnet at the patient's bedside in the event that electrical interference leads to pacemaker inhibition and bradycardia [48]. The recommendations for patients with an ICD are to turn off the detection mode of the ICD during ECT, perform continuous ECG monitoring throughout the treatment with careful attention to grounding, and place resuscitative equipment by the patient's bedside in the event that external defibrillation is necessary [48].

7.3 Respiratory Complications

7.3.1 Prolonged Apnea

Case reports shows that prolonged apnea occurs during ECT procedure in patients with butyrylcholinesterase deficiency, which is a metabolic disorder characterized by prolonged apnea after the use of certain anesthetic drugs including the muscle relaxants succinylcholine or mivacurium and other ester local anesthetics [67]. The short duration of action of succinylcholine is due to its rapid hydrolysis by butyrylcholinesterase to succinylmonocholine and choline, and butyrylcholinesterase is synthesized by the liver and found in plasma [68]. Another case report showed prolonged apnea during an ECT procedure with succinylcholine, in which the patient was also being treated with a topical organophosphate anticholinesterase, echothiophate iodide (phospholine iodide), for glaucoma. The increased duration of action of succinylcholine resulted from low levels of serum cholinesterase caused by the organophosphate [69]. Other factors that have been described as lowering butyrylcholinesterase activity are liver disease, advanced age, malnutrition, pregnancy, burns, oral contraceptives, monoamine oxidase inhibitors, echothiophate, cytotoxic drugs, neoplastic disease, tetrahydroaminacrine, hexafluorenium, and metoclopramide [68]. Attention is called to other drugs that directly or indirectly (by lowering serum cholinesterase) interact with succinylcholine chloride, resulting in prolonged apnea [69]. Before the ECT procedure, airway assessment is important in each patient.

7.3.2 Pulmonary Embolism

Physical restraint during seclusion and the use of antipsychotic agents can be risk factors for deep vein thrombosis (DVT) [70]. Catatonic patients often experience prolonged inactivity and dehydration and thus are prone to venous stasis, leading to life-threatening DVT and pulmonary embolism (PE) [71, 72]. Although PE as a complication of ECT has been reported [73–77], ECT can be considered in this population based on a risk-benefit analysis, and it is important to involve the family in obtaining informed consent. Clinebell et al. [72] reviewed and summarized the guidelines for DVT/PE prophylaxis.

7.3.3 Aspiration Pneumonia

Pulmonary aspiration following ECT was not uncommon before the era of muscle relaxants (before 1961), but after the introduction of these agents, aspiration following ECT was not reported again until 1988 [78, 79]. General anesthesia with muscle relaxation has made ECT safer [78–80]. Nevertheless, there are some case reports of episodes of gastric aspiration associated with pneumonia and subsequent acute respiratory distress syndrome following ECT: both patients were found to have loss of gastric muscle tone (gastroparesis) [78, 79]. These findings suggest that candidates for ECT should be screened for gastroparesis, in addition to other well-recognized conditions that are associated with an increased risk of complications during or following ECT.

Although another case report by Tecoult and Nathan [81] claimed that ECT is not a low-risk procedure because of the particularly high rate of life-threatening respiratory complications such as aspiration pneumonitis, hypoxia, laryngospasm, and bronchospasm in their patients, Swartz [82] argued that this conclusion was an extrapolation from these authors' own experience, and also their ECT procedure included several peculiarities that undermined their claim, particularly the omission of a muscle paralysis agent such as succinylcholine, with Meignan [83] and Wild et al. [84] both counterclaiming that this omission explained much of the morbidity.

Abrams [80], who is a psychiatrist, recommends that ECT candidates with concurrent disorders (e.g., diabetes mellitus, hypothyroidism, amyloidosis, and scleroderma) judged to put them at high risk for gastroparesis, which is a common disorder that produces symptoms of gastric retention in the absence of physical obstruction [85], should have a careful gastrointestinal history taken followed by a gastrointestinal series or radionucleotide gastric emptying study, if indicated. Abrams [80] further commented that the only sure way to prevent vomiting – and aspiration of gastric contents – in patients with documented gastroparesis is to remove the stomach contents by nasogastric tube suction before induction of anesthesia. However, Kurnutala et al. [78], who are anesthesiologists, insisted that patients are not usually considered to have a "full stomach" with depression, even though there is the possibility of depression-induced gastroparesis [85], and depression is not usually associated with aspiration pneumonitis [85]. Furthermore, they advocated that if every patient with major depression were considered to have a "full stomach," all patients would need to be intubated with a rapid sequence induction for their ECT, and subjecting every patient with a history of depression and ongoing antidepressant use to gastric motility studies before interventions requiring brief anesthesia is unrealistic and introduces its own set of costs and risks [78].

The *Practice Guidelines for Preoperative Fasting and the Use of Pharmacologic Agents to Reduce the Risk of Pulmonary Aspiration* published by the ASA in 1999 relaxed the traditional policy of NPO (nothing by mouth) to permit the ingestion of clear liquids up to 2 h before elective procedures requiring anesthesia. In the updated guidelines published in 2011, 6 h of fasting following the ingestion of solid food is recommended, with ingestion of fried or fatty foods requiring a longer fast of 8 h or more because such foods may prolong gastric emptying time [86, 87]. These recommendations are not intended for women in labor and are applicable only to healthy patients undergoing elective procedures [86]. The recommended fasting times do not guarantee complete gastric emptying and, further, are applicable to patients of any age [86]. Recommended clear liquids include water, pulpless fruit juices, carbonated beverages, clear tea, and black coffee [86]. When determining an appropriate fasting period, the amount of milk ingested must be taken into account because the gastric emptying time of nonhuman milk is prolonged, similar to that of solids. A light meal is generally considered to be toast and clear liquids [86]. Meals that include fried or fatty foods or meat may prolong gastric emptying time, and additional fasting time (e.g., 8 h or more) may be needed in these cases [86]. Thus, to determine an appropriate fasting period, it is necessary to consider both the amount and type of food ingested [86]. The ASA guidelines do not specifically address chewing gum, hard candies, and smoking; however, the European Society of Anaesthesiology guidelines do not consider it necessary to delay the induction of anesthesia if foods such as gum and hard candies have been consumed immediately before the procedure [88]. Although not recommended by the ASA guidelines [86, 87], routine use of drugs to prevent aspiration pneumonitis may be worthwhile in patients with specific risk factors for aspiration. Such factors include a full stomach, hiatal hernia, symptomatic gastroesophageal reflux disease, morbid obesity, diabetic gastroparesis, presence of a nasogastric tube, or pregnancy [86, 87]. Prophylaxis against aspiration can decrease gastric volume and increase the pH of the gastric fluid. Drugs commonly used include nonparticulate antacids (e.g., Bicitra), promotility drugs (e.g., metoclopramide), and H_2-receptor antagonists, which can be used alone or in combination [87].

Berrios and Sage [89] conducted a prospective study into the more objective clinical characteristics of a cohort of fast-breakers: of 81 patients undergoing ECT during a period of 24 months, 21 had eaten or drunk something against medical advice shortly before ECT was performed. Compared with control subjects, the fast-breakers were less often married, were more likely to be detained under a section of the Mental Health Act, had an unfavorable view of ECT, and often had not given consent for ECT. Fast-breaking was more likely to occur after four or more ECTs. There was a significant correlation among the fast-breakers between age and (a) the number of previous ECTs and (b) the treatment at which the fast-break occurred. The more drugs the patient was taking, the more likely it was that the fast would be broken early in the course of ECT. They recommended that patients meeting the criteria mentioned above be subject to special observation and given special counseling before and during any course of ECT.

7.3.4 Pulmonary Edema

Pulmonary edema after ECT is an infrequent but serious complication requiring timely recognition and management to avoid significant morbidity and mortality [90]. Types of pulmonary edema include negative-pressure pulmonary edema [91–93], neurogenic pulmonary edema [90, 94–97], cardiogenic pulmonary edema, aspiration, and others.

Three cases of negative-pressure pulmonary edema after ECT have been reported. One case occurred when, on awakening from her fourth treatment, the patient began coughing violently and developed laryngospasm; physical examination revealed bilateral crepitation at the lung bases, and a small amount of pink frothy sputum was observed [91]. Her chest radiograph demonstrated mild pulmonary edema, and she recovered after diuresis with 20 mg of furosemide and overnight observation [91]. Another case occurred in a man with asthma treated with clenbuterol hydrochloride, a β_2 stimulant. About 10 min after receiving esmolol, a short-acting β-adrenergic blocker, to address hypertension and tachycardia after his eighth ECT treatment, his blood oxygen saturation fell [92]. He had a small amount of bloody sputum, and chest auscultation revealed coarse crackles. Chest x-ray showed peripheral infiltrates, and he recovered after treatment with intravenous hydrocortisone [92]. The authors concluded that the pulmonary edema may have been triggered by esmolol-induced bronchospasm, thiopental-induced laryngospasm, or possibly from redistribution of the blood volume to the pulmonary vasculature enhanced by the activity of the clenbuterol [92]. The third case was of a man with FG syndrome [98], which is a rare X-linked multiple congenital anomaly-cognitive impairment disorder, and the acute pulmonary edema likely was precipitated by the patient generating a large inspiratory effort due to inadequate muscular paralysis either against a closed glottis or an airway obstructed by the bite block pushing his tongue into the posterior oropharyngeal space [93]. It is also possible that mechanical irritation from the bite block caused laryngospasm, thus reinforcing the upper airway obstruction [93].

Acute neurogenic pulmonary edema can result from almost any type of central nervous system insult, including stroke, trauma, hemorrhage, drugs, or seizure [97], and five cases of neurogenic pulmonary edema after ECT have been reported

[90, 94–97]. A small study of 12 people undergoing ECT discovered one case of subclinical pulmonary edema on posttreatment chest radiography [95]. Pulmonary edema often has been reported as a complication of epileptic seizures and was found at autopsy in more than 86 % of epileptics who died unexpectedly [99]. Although the modern practice of muscle paralysis camouflages the induced seizure, the goal of ECT is to produce bilateral convulsions similar to that occurring during a spontaneous generalized convulsion, and thus, some degree of pulmonary edema following ECT may be more common than previously expected [97]. Although a multifactorial model is likely to explain the pathophysiology of neurogenic pulmonary edema, animal studies suggest that "neurocentric foci" in the hypothalamus control sympathetic tracts leaving the brain [97, 100]. Irritation of these foci from trauma or otherwise (e.g., ECT) can result in a systemic sympathetic response leading to pulmonary edema [97]. Pulmonary edema can be induced in animals by intracisternal injection of thrombin and fibrinogen [101]. Within 2 min of injection, there are marked increases in intracranial pressure, α- and β-adrenergic stimulation, and systemic vascular resistance [102]. During this time of intense α-adrenergic stimulation in the peripheral vessels, blood is quickly redistributed from the higher-resistance systemic circuit to the lower-resistance pulmonary vasculature [103], and increased pulmonary capillary wedge pressure unbalances Starling's forces leading to pulmonary edema [104]. Furthermore, cardiovascular dysfunction also may contribute to neurogenic pulmonary edema [97]. Left ventricular hypokinesia and regional wall motion abnormalities associated with ECG changes suggestive of myocardial ischemia have also been demonstrated during the blood pressure and heart rate elevation occurring with ECT [57]. ECT causes increased myocardial oxygen demand, which may lead to transient ischemia and myocardial dysfunction [94]. Diastolic dysfunction also may play a role and has been implicated in acute pulmonary edema associated with hypertension after ECT [105].

7.3.5 Bronchospasm

There are some case reports of bronchospasm following ECT [81, 106]; however, not every patient had a history of asthma or chronic obstructive pulmonary disease (COPD). The incidence of wheezing is higher in asthmatic patients receiving thiopental for induction than in those given propofol, and thiopental itself does not cause bronchospasm, but it may inadequately suppress upper airway reflexes [107]. Nonetheless, for the asthma or COPD patient, assessment of the severity of the disease and therapy before the ECT procedure is very important.

Management of patients with asthma attacks and/or exacerbations of acute COPD during ECT is similar and follows recommended guidelines [108–111]. First-line treatment, in addition to the administration of oxygen to prevent hypoxemia, includes an inhaled β-adrenergic agonist combined with an anticholinergic agent such as albuterol or salbutamol plus ipratropium, which can be delivered by metered-dose inhaler or nebulized aerosol. Frequently, a systemic corticosteroid such as methylprednisolone administered in an IV bolus dose of 60–125 mg is often used [111]. Particularly, intravenous β-adrenergic agonists such as epinephrine injected in a 100 to 200 μg IV bolus dose can be helpful during exacerbations of life-threatening asthma or COPD. Endotracheal intubation is also warranted in patients with impending or actual respiratory arrest with ketamine being the drug of choice because of its bronchodilating properties [111]. Other conditions, such as pneumonia, pneumothorax, anaphylaxis, and pulmonary embolism, can also increase the severity of hypoxemia, and the ECT team must be aware of these conditions [111].

7.4 Prolonged Seizures

Most seizures are self-limiting, lasting less than 2 min [112]. In rare instances, however, persistent seizure activity (prolonged seizure and status epilepticus) or a recurrence of seizure activity (tardive seizures) may occur [112, 113]. The incidence is thought to be 1 % of treatments in adults [3]. Seizures with motor and/or electroencephalography (EEG) manifestations persisting for more than 180 s should be considered "prolonged" [114]. The presence of prolonged seizures may be apparent only with EEG monitoring, which is especially useful [112, 114] because most seizures are undetectable by motor observation alone [112]. Furthermore, the ECT practitioner should determine whether seizure activity is ongoing as opposed to EEG artifact [114]. Prolonged seizures are particularly likely to occur in one of the following circumstances: (1) at the first treatment, (2) during benzodiazepine withdrawal, (3) in patients in whom proconvulsant medications (e.g., caffeine, theophylline) and lithium are used concurrently, or (4) in patients who have epilepsy or preexisting paroxysmal EEG activity [112, 113]. Prolonged seizures should be terminated pharmacologically with an anesthetic agent or benzodiazepine after 3 min of sustained seizure activity [112, 114]. Seizures can be terminated by intravenous administration of either a repeat dose of the anesthetic agent (e.g., methohexital, thiopental, or propofol [115]) or a short-acting benzodiazepine (e.g., midazolam 1–2 mg), and if after 2 more minutes the seizure is still not aborted, the dose should be repeated [112]. If the patient continues to experience seizure activity, immediate neurology consultation should be obtained, blood gases and electrolytes should be checked, and lorazepam (2–4 mg IV over 1 min) or diazepam (5–10 mg IV) should be given [112]. During and immediately after prolonged seizures, it is important that the patient continues to receive adequate oxygenation, and this may be accomplished via positive-pressure ventilation or by the placement of an endotracheal tube [112, 114]. Adequate muscular relaxation should also be ensured [112]. ECT should be resumed only after correcting any treatable conditions known to increase the likelihood of prolonged seizures and assessing the applicable risk/benefit ratio [114]. The APA recommends that each facility should have policies outlining the steps to be taken to terminate prolonged seizures and status epilepticus [116].

7.5 Central Nervous System Complications

7.5.1 Overview of Space-Occupying or Intracranial Vascular Lesions

Large increases in cerebral blood flow and intracranial pressure occur as direct effects of the ECT stimulus and seizure [9, 117]. ECT in patients with intracranial vascular masses must be approached cautiously because patients may be at risk of aneurysmal rupture following the temporary rise in blood pressure during or after seizure activity [7, 118]. Because increased intracranial pressure might lead to herniation and death, intracranial masses or space-occupying lesions have been considered contraindications to ECT for quite some time [48]. Although in early case reports of such patients, the reported neurologic outcomes were poor, these studies were probably subject to selection bias, since neurologic deterioration after ECT prompted diagnosis of an intracranial lesion in all but 1 of the 35 patients [48, 119]. More recently, patients with known intracranial lesions with normal neurologic examinations and little to no edema or presence of a mass on neuroimaging were reported to have safely undergone ECT [48, 120]. Neuroimaging is recommended in patients with abnormal neurologic examinations or known masses to search for possible changes consistent with increased intracranial pressure. Successful ECT was reported in a patient with an intracranial lesion and surrounding edema [121]. Assessment of the safety of ECT in such high-risk patients will require additional prospective study [48]

The evidence regarding the safety of ECT in patients with intracranial vascular lesions is limited. The APA lists this as a high-risk condition because the increased rate-pressure product during and after the seizure could lead to aneurysmal rupture [122]. There appear to be no published reports of ruptured cerebral aneurysms due to ECT. In the largest case series to date, there were no complications in six patients with intracranial vascular lesions (in all cases the lesions were <10 mm in diameter) who underwent ECT [123]. Before ECT is performed in patients with intracranial masses or vascular lesions, the neurologist, neurosurgeon, or both, as well as the anesthesiologist, should participate in the evaluation of the patient and in the process of informed consent.

7.5.2 Recent Cerebral Infarction and Hemorrhage

Limited data are available on preexisting cerebrovascular disease in patients undergoing ECT. However, one study involving patients with a history of strokes reported no lasting neurologic complications following ECT [48, 124]. In patients with a history of recent or acute stroke, changes in intracranial pressure and cerebral blood flow caused by ECT may place the patient at risk of ischemia or hemorrhage [48]. Of the 14 patients studied in this report, five underwent ECT within 1 month poststroke, all without major complications [48, 124]. As with poststroke patients undergoing noncardiac surgery, delay of ECT at least until 1 month after the acute stroke is suggested [48, 125]. As well, minimization of both hypertension and hypotension through tight blood pressure control may reduce the respective risks of bleeding and additional ischemia [48].

7.5.3 Subdural Hematoma

Acute or chronic subdural hematoma is rare, but it can be a serious complication following ECT [126–128]. It is important to investigate patients with neurological signs and symptoms of subdural hematoma following ECT, and a computed tomography or magnetic resonance imaging scan should be performed as appropriate. The anticipation of complications along with their early diagnosis and treatment are the most important factors in delivering comprehensive ECT [127].

7.6 Headache

The incidence of headache after ECT is likely higher than generally recognized [129]. Although many patients do not spontaneously report headache, when specifically asked, roughly half of the patients may report some degree of discomfort [129]. Headaches after ECT have a specific "throbbing" frontal character [7]. Some patients complain of short bouts of headaches that are definitely mild to moderate in intensity, and rarely, other patients report migraine-like headaches [130]. These headaches react well to acetylsalicylic acid, acetaminophen, or other anti-inflammatory agents such as ibuprofen [130, 131]. However, the migraine-type headaches usually do not respond to these treatment modalities, and some authors mention the use of acute antimigraine agents such as sumatriptan given intranasally [132]. In addition, others studied migraine-prevention therapies such as β-adrenergic blockers, valproic acid, topiramate, and mirtazapine, all of which showed positive effects [130]. A different approach was to prescribe the prophylactic use of ketorolac (for headache or myalgias) or caffeine given as intravenous caffeine sodium benzoate, this having several potential beneficial effects including seizure prolongation and headache prophylaxis [133]. Another prophylactic study showed good results with sumatriptan given before ECT [134]. The pathophysiological mechanism of ECT-induced headaches is unknown. The literature regarding ECT administered to depressed patients shows that changes in serotonin levels are linked to treatment efficacy. This feature is common to the action of antidepressant drugs as modulators of 5-HT receptors. ECT induces upregulation of 5-HT_2 receptors, whereas antidepressant drugs cause downregulation. This sensitization secondary to the 5-HT_2 upregulation might be responsible for the generation of headaches [135]. Routine preventive treatment of post-ECT headache may not be necessary in older patients without a history of severe headache, but it might be of benefit in younger patients and those who have previously experienced more severe post-ECT headache [129].

7.7 Fracture and Dislocation

The tonic-clonic convulsions associated with ECT can result in injuries such as limb fractures and compression fractures of the vertebral bodies [136, 137].

7.7.1 Fracture of Vertebrae and Spinal Cord Compression

Although fractures of the vertebrae and spinal cord compression following ECT are rare, they may occur in a compromised patient [138]. Vertebral compression fracture affects older individuals, predominantly women with osteoporosis [139]. Before the use of general anesthesia and muscle relaxation, compression fractures were a common occurrence during ECT [139]. However, with the advent of modern anesthesia techniques in ECT, vertebral compression fractures are now a rare complication [139], and there is a case report of the safe administration of ECT to a depressed patient with severe, unstable cervical spine disease [140]. Nevertheless, careful attention must be paid to muscular relaxation, particularly in high-risk patients with osteoporosis [139]; compression fractures of the spine should not occur with adequate muscle relaxation [141].

7.7.2 Fracture

Although the introduction of anesthesia, especially neuromuscular blockade, can mitigate tonic-clonic motor activity and reduce the physical and physiologic trauma associated with uncontrolled tetanic muscle contractions [136, 137], fractures are a known side effect of ECT. In any patient with osteoporosis, an appropriate dose of a muscle relaxant should be administered to prevent fractures. Although bone injury while undergoing ECT is thought to be rare, there are case reports of fracture of the neck of the femur during treatment [142, 143], and there is a case report of a patient with rheumatoid arthritis who suffered a fractured humerus that required surgical repair (although use of succinylcholine was unclear) [81]. Further, a recent paper reported on a patient who fractured his ulna after hitting his arm violently on a bed rail during an ECT-induced seizure, and lack of muscle relaxation was noted as the root cause of this event [4]. More complete neuromuscular blockade may be acceptable in high-risk patients who may be more likely to suffer fractures if the degree of neuromuscular blockade is underestimated [9].

7.7.3 Dislocation

Dislocation of the shoulder and pelvic girdle secondary to seizures is a known complication of ECT [144–147]. However, dislocations should not occur with adequate muscle relaxation [141].

7.8 Postictal Agitation, Delirium, and Confusional States

Postictal agitation is a relatively frequent clinical complication with ECT [11], reported in up to 7 % of ECT sessions [148], in 10 % of patients who undergo a course of ECT [82], and in up to 12 % of patients with delirium [149]. Clinical characteristics of agitation in the setting of ECT include disorientation, motor restlessness, aimless movements, nonresponse to verbal commands, panic-like behavior or fear, and even attempts to leave the recovery room [11]. An episode can last from 5 min to 1 h or more [11, 150]. It is important for the clinician to keep in mind that what initially seems like agitation may be nonconvulsive epileptic activity, and therefore the EEG tracing needs to be assessed promptly to rule out prolonged seizure as a cause of postictal agitation [11]. If prolonged seizure is in doubt, intravenous antiseizure medication needs to be administered without delay [11]. Either way, emergent management of postictal agitation with short-acting benzodiazepines such as midazolam and lorazepam represents a first-line intervention that can serve both purposes [11, 151]. A good second-line option is intravenous haloperidol [11, 151], and boluses of propofol [11, 151] or methohexital can also be effective for severe postictal agitation with the advantage of these drugs being immediately at hand if they were used as the anesthetic agent. Nevertheless, postictal agitation is often easily managed nonpharmacologically [151].

7.9 Increased Intraocular Pressure

Recent reports suggest that patients with glaucoma have a higher prevalence of depression in contrast to control subjects. Taking this into consideration, it is expected that more and more patients with glaucoma will require treatment for their depression, and at least some of these patients with severe depression may require ECT [152]. It is known that ECT causes a transient rise in intraocular pressure in patients with and without glaucoma [152–154]. However, it is not known whether such a rise is clinically important [153]. Narrow-angle glaucoma, which is invariably associated with symptoms, is an ophthalmologic emergency requiring treatment before ECT should be undertaken [155]. However, the APA notes that no reports have been published of such patients being referred for ECT [156]. In the past, acute or evolving retinal detachment has also been considered a substantial risk of ECT, but no reports of such problems have been published [156].

7.10 Myalgias and Muscle Soreness

Posttreatment myalgia also seems to be quite common after ECT [129] and may be associated with the use of succinylcholine as a muscle relaxant [129]. Succinylcholine is generally used in ECT because of its rapid onset and short duration of action, despite an incidence of muscle pain after administration that has been reported to vary widely, from 0.2 to 89 % [129]. It is postulated that this pain is secondary to damage produced in muscle by the unsynchronized contraction of adjacent muscle fibers just before the onset of paralysis [157]. This concept has been substantiated by the findings of myoglobinemia and increased serum creatine kinase following succinylcholine administration [158]. Myalgias are significantly more intense after the first ECT treatment than after later treatments [129], and younger subjects are more often affected, perhaps because of their greater relative muscle mass [129]. No relation has been found between myalgia and either observed motor seizure vigor or fasciculations [129, 159].

7.11 Injury to the Mouth (Including Dental and Tongue Injury)

During the electrical stimulation in ECT, clenching of the jaw may occur as a result of direct stimulation of the masseter muscle, and the most commonly reported adverse events related to ECT are injury to the mouth (including dental and tongue injuries) and problems related to paralysis (no muscle relaxation) [4]. Injury to the teeth and other oral structure remains a risk in ECT despite the use of muscle relaxants [160]. The teeth are liable to excessive stress because the electrodes are placed on the temporal muscle, quite close to the masseter muscle [161]. Biting pressure in a conscious individual is controlled by a feedback mechanism so that excessive strain is avoided, but an anesthetized patient does not experience such feedback [161]. Furthermore, it is likely that patients undergoing ECT will have a diseased or heavily restored dentition that is more sensitive to damage [161]. In addition to the loosening of teeth, there is also a danger of aspirating loose teeth and damage to the masticator muscles [161]. The soft oral tissues may also be damaged by invaginating the lips or by biting the cheeks, and sometimes such damage necessitates delaying subsequent ECT treatments, thus adding greatly to the patient's distress and discomfort [162]. To prevent these complications, various types of gags, mouth guards and dental protectors have been described in the literature [81, 161]. Both incorrect bite block placement and failure to use a bite block can be a cause of injury [4]. Broken teeth should not occur with adequate muscle relaxation [141]. Because of the muscular contractions, dental appliances (e.g., dentures) should be removed before treatment [163].

7.12 Nausea and Vomiting

The incidence of post-ECT nausea was reported to range from 1 to 23 % [164]; however, as with headache, methodologic issues make the true incidence difficult to quantify [164]. Severe post-ECT headaches and nausea are two of the reasons why some patients discontinue their course of ECT [165]. Although the underlying pathophysiologic cause of post-ECT headaches and nausea remains unclear [165], nausea may occur secondary to headache or to treatment of the headache with narcotics, particularly in patients with a vascular-type headache [164]. Nausea may also occur independently as a side effect of anesthesia because of the withdrawal or institution of psychotropic medications or by other unknown mechanisms [164]. When nausea accompanies the headache, the primary treatment should focus on the relief of the headache as outlined above. Otherwise, post-ECT nausea is typically well controlled with dopamine-blocking agents such as the phenothiazine derivatives (e.g., prochlorperazine), butyrophenones (haloperidol, droperidol), trimethobenzamide, or metoclopramide [164]. If the nausea does not respond to these treatments or if adverse effects preclude the use of dopaminergic antagonists, the serotonin 5-HT_3 receptor antagonists ondansetron and dolasetron may be useful alternatives [164, 165]. Some cases of nausea or vomiting may be associated with the anesthetic agent used, which can be changed if necessary after discussion with the anesthesiologist [3]. Mirtazapine is an antidepressant that possesses antagonizing effects on postsynaptic serotonins 5-HT_2 and 5-HT_3, and there is a published case series suggesting that mirtazapine may be an optional treatment for ECT-induced headaches and nausea [165].

7.13 Salivation

Seizure activity causes an initial parasympathetic discharge manifested by bradycardia, occasional asystole, premature atrial and ventricular contractions, or a combination of these abnormalities, and hypotension and salivation can also occur as side effect of ECT [9]. Anticholinergic premedication is common in ECT, and the main reason an anticholinergic given is to prevent vagally mediated bradyarrhythmias. It also reduces airway secretions [166, 167]. Glycopyrrolate or atropine can be chosen as anticholinergic agents [167, 168]. It is helpful to know that clozapine was found to be superior to traditional neuroleptics in the treatment of refractory schizophrenia, and clozapine-induced hypersalivation is a potential source of aspiration in the delirious state, and therefore, careful monitoring and preventive measures are advised [169].

7.14 Hyperglycemia

The effect of ECT on blood glucose is unpredictable because of changes in diet, appetite, and energy level that may result from ECT. Individual ECT treatments raise blood glucose levels in patients with diabetes to the same degree as in patients without diabetes [48] because norepinephrine and epinephrine increase immediately after ECT, and epinephrine levels decrease more rapidly thereafter [9]. Glucose homeostasis is variably affected by ECT [9]. Improvement in the control of non-insulin-dependent diabetes is generally noted, whereas hyperglycemia may be seen when the diabetes is insulin dependent [9]. There is one case report of hyperglycemia in a patient with no previous history of diabetes [170]. It is recommended that blood glucose levels be measured before and after ECT treatment, that short-acting insulin be available to treat elevations in blood glucose level, and that ECT be performed early in the morning if possible [48].

7.15 Allergic Reactions

During the ECT procedure, several drugs such as anticholinergic agents (glycopyrrolate and atropine [167, 168]), intravenous anesthetics (methohexital, thiopental, propofol, ketamine, and etomidate) or volatile anesthetics (sevoflurane [20]), and neuromuscular blockade agents (succinylcholine, mivacurium, atracurium, cisatracurium, and rocuronium) are commonly used, and the ECT team should know the various side effects of these drugs. Minor drug reactions such as a skin rash are not an uncommon occurrence, and major reactions such as anaphylactic shock occur much less often [171].

The incidence of anaphylaxis and anaphylactoid reactions during anesthesia is very difficult to estimate but has been calculated to range from 1 in 3,500 to 1 in 13,000 cases [172–175]. A report from Australia estimated the incidence to be between 1 in 10,000 and 1 in 20,000 [174–176], whereas a more recent report from Norway estimated the incidence to be 1 in 6,000 [174, 177]. Muscle relaxants are associated with the most frequent incidence of anaphylaxis, and natural rubber latex has emerged as the second most common cause of anaphylaxis [174]. Another paper showed the agents involved in anaphylactic reactions during anesthesia ($n = 518$) between January 1, 1999, and December 31, 2000, in France [178], and the most common causes of anaphylaxis were neuromuscular blocking agents ($n = 306$, 58.2 %), latex ($n = 88$, 16.7 %), and antibiotics ($n = 79$, 15.1 %), with rocuronium ($n = 132$, 43.1 %) and succinylcholine ($n = 69$, 22.6 %) being the most frequently incriminated neuromuscular blocking agents [178]. A recent paper analyzed the rate of anaphylaxis to neuromuscular blocking drugs over a 10-year period in the only specialized diagnostic center in Western Australia, and rocuronium was responsible for 56 %, succinylcholine for 21 %, and vecuronium for 11 % of the cases of anaphylaxis [179]. Furthermore, this paper concluded that after accounting for usage rate, rocuronium had a three-fold increased risk of IgE-mediated anaphylaxis compared with vecuronium [179]. The most recently published paper (2014), which is a retrospective, observational cohort study of intraoperative anaphylaxis to neuromuscular blocking drugs at two hospitals in Auckland, New Zealand, between 2006 and 2012, showed that the incidence of anaphylaxis was 1 in 22,451 new patient exposures for atracurium, 1 in 2080 for succinylcholine, and 1 in 2499 for rocuronium [180].

Although rare, IgE-mediated hypersensitivity reactions may lead to death, even when appropriately treated, with a mortality ranging from 3.5 % in Australia [181, 182], 4.7 % in Japan [182, 183], and 10 % in the United Kingdom [182, 184].

The treatment of anaphylaxis involves epinephrine to interrupt the cascade of profound vasodilation and significant vascular leak [171], and if possible, the offending drug should be removed or stopped [171], with oxygenation administered as well. Epinephrine (10- to 100-μg bolus if not pulseless; 1- to 3-mg bolus if pulseless; and infusion at 4–10 μg/min) and vasopressin (0.5- to 2-unit bolus if not pulseless; 40-unit bolus if pulseless) can be used to support the blood pressure, while intravenous steroids (e.g., hydrocortisone 50–150 mg) and intravenous antihistamines (e.g., diphenhydramine 50 mg as an H_1 blocker and famotidine

20 mg as an H_2 blocker) are administered to further attenuate the response [171]. Intravenous fluid administration is essential secondary to the vascular leak [171]. CPR and ACLS should be instituted immediately if there is no pulse [171]. In the event of complete cardiovascular collapse, much larger doses of epinephrine may be required [171]. The ECT team should always be prepared to treat anaphylactic or anaphylactoid responses.

7.16 Bladder and Gastric Rupture

7.16.1 Bladder Rupture

There is a case report of bladder rupture following tonic-clonic seizures [185], and also there are some case reports showing bladder rupture after ECT [186, 187]. Following ECT, one of the patients had a history of prostatism [186], and another patient, who was taking amitriptyline 150 mg/day, had failed to void before treatment [187]. Schizophrenic patients have been reported to have detrusor hyperreflexia [186], and these cases amply support the standard recommendation for patients to void their bladder before undergoing ECT [188]. The presence of hematuria, absence of urinary output, and increasing abdominal distension are highly suggestive of a ruptured urinary bladder [185].

7.16.2 Gastric Rupture

There is one case report of gastric rupture following ECT for which the mechanism of gastric rupture was thought to be as follows [189]. Most likely, during mask ventilation, air was forced into the stomach, probably because of poor mask ventilation technique or inadequate positioning, causing mild gastric inflation, a common complication that often goes undetected [189]. Because the patient's muscles were likely not completely relaxed during ECT administration, the induced convulsion produced strong contractions of the abdominal muscles, and as a result, the distended stomach ruptured like a balloon [189].

Diagnostic features of gastric rupture consist of severe upper abdominal pain followed by tympanic abdominal distension, abdominal rigidity, subcutaneous emphysema, and shock [189]. Rupture of the stomach is a rare but serious event, mostly caused by an ulcer or trauma, and if gastric rupture is suspected, a chest and abdomen x-ray should be performed, preferably with the patient sitting up, to detect free subphrenic air [189]. All patients require operative treatment by laparotomy and subsequent closure of the rupture [189].

Van Schaik et al. [189] suggest the following recommendations. First, during the pre-ECT screening, special attention should be given to the recognition of risk factors predisposing to gastric rupture such as gastric ulcer and the use of nonsteroidal anti-inflammatory drugs, and second, during ventilation, gastric inflation and difficult ventilation are important potential risk factors, especially if complete muscle relaxation is doubtful [189]. Both psychiatrists and anesthesiologists should be aware of this rare but serious complication [189] even though complications involving abdominal organs are very rare in ECT procedures.

7.17 Other Complications

Other complications such as treatment-emergent mania and cognitive side effects may not be noted by the ECT anesthesiologist because they occur after ECT treatment. However, ECT psychiatrists should be aware of the facts relating to these side effects.

7.17.1 Treatment-Emergent Mania

As with pharmacologic antidepressant treatments, a small minority of patients with depression or those in mixed affective states switch into states of hypomania or mania during the ECT course [190]. Although this reaction is rare, patients with bipolar disorder may be the most likely to show this effect [164]. This switch may be managed by either continuing the ECT course or stopping ECT and administering an antimanic agent [1]. The action taken usually depends on whether overt mania is present, in which case it is preferable (although also counterintuitive to some degree) to continue the ECT [1].

7.17.2 Cognitive Side Effects, Cognitive Changes, and Memory Impairment

Cognitive changes are often the most notable and most distressing side effects of ECT [1], but a detailed discussion of these side effects is beyond the scope of this article. Nevertheless, the clinician, and especially ECT psychiatrists, should be aware of several facts concerning cognitive changes [1, 191]. First, depressive episodes themselves are often accompanied by profound cognitive changes, which are sometimes severe enough to present as dementia (pseudodementia) [1]. In such cases, a successful response to ECT may actually be associated with at least a subjective improvement in cognitive status [1]. Second, cognitive change is not equivalent to structural brain damage, and extensive research has found no relation between ECT and brain damage [1]. Three types of cognitive impairment may be observed with ECT: postictal disorientation, interictal confusion, and amnesia (anterograde [i.e., inability to retain new memories] and retrograde [i.e., loss of recall of events before treatment] memory disturbances or both) [1, 48]. The methods used in ECT administration have a profound effect on the nature and magnitude of cognitive deficits. For example, in general, bilateral electrode placement, sine wave stimulation, high electrode dosage relative to seizure threshold, closely spaced treatments, larger numbers of treatments, and high dosage of barbiturate anesthetic agents are each independently associated with more intense cognitive side effects compared with right unilateral electrode placement, brief pulse waveform, lower electrical intensity, more widely spaced treatments, fewer treatments, and lower dosage of barbiturate anesthesia [191, 192]. The first large-scale prospective study of objective cognitive outcomes of patients treated with ECT showed advanced age to be associated with an increased severity of cognitive deficits [193]. Most cognitive deficits except for loss of psychomotor function and autobiographical memory resolve within 6 months after the initiation of treatment [48]. In contrast, in a systematic review of patients' perceptions of ECT, 29–55 % of the patients with depression reported persistent memory loss for more than 6 months after ECT [48, 194].

References

1. Mankad MV, Weiner RD. Adverse effects. In: Mankad MV, Beyer JL, Weiner RD, Krystal AD, editors. Clinical manual of electroconvulsive therapy. Arlington: American Psychiatric Publishing, Inc.; 2010. p. 139–48.
2. Abrams R. The mortality rate with ECT. Convuls Ther. 1997;13:125–7.
3. Consoli A, De Carvalho W, Cohen D. Side effect of ECT. In: Ghaziuddin N, Walter G, editors. Electroconvulsive therapy in children and adolescents. New York: Oxford University Press; 2013. p. 140–60.
4. Watts BV, Groft A, Bagian JP, Mills PD. An examination of mortality and other adverse events related to electroconvulsive therapy using a national adverse event report system. J ECT. 2011;27:105–8.
5. Shiwach RS, Reid WH, Carmody TJ. An analysis of reported deaths following electroconvulsive therapy in Texas, 1993–1998. Psychiatr Serv. 2001;52:1095–7.
6. Nuttall GA, Bowersox MR, Douglass SB, McDonald J, Rasmussen LJ, Decker PA, Oliver Jr WC, Rasmussen KG. Morbidity and mortality in the use of electroconvulsive therapy. J ECT. 2004;20:237–41.
7. American Psychiatric Association. The practice of electroconvulsive therapy: recommendations for treatment, training, and priveleging, A task force report of the American Psychiatric Association. 2nd ed. Washington, DC: American Psychiatric Association; 2001.
8. Tomac TA, Rummans TA, Pileggi TS, Li H. Safety and efficacy of electroconvulsive therapy in patients over age 85. Am J Geriatr Psychiatry. 1997;5:126–30.
9. Stensrud PE. Anesthesia at remote locations. In: Miller RD, editor. Miller's anesthesia, vol. 2. 7th ed. Philadelphia: Churchill Livingstone Elsevier; 2010. p. 2477–9.
10. Boere E, Birkenhager TK, Groenland TH, van den Broek WW. Beta-blocking agents during electroconvulsive therapy: a review. Br J Anaesth. 2014;113:43–51.
11. Cristancho MA, Alici Y, Augoustides JG, O'Reardon JP. Uncommon but serious complications associated with electroconvulsive therapy: recognition and management for the clinician. Curr Psychiatry Rep. 2008;10:474–80.
12. Bhat SK, Acosta D, Swartz CM. Postictal asystole during ECT. J ECT. 2002;18:103–6.
13. Robinson M, Lighthall G. Asystole during successive electroconvulsive therapy sessions: a report of two cases. J Clin Anesth. 2004;16:210–3.
14. Welch CA. Medical evaluation before electroconvulsive therapy. N Engl J Med. 2009;360:2791–2; author reply 2.
15. Bryson EO, Kellner CH, Ahle GM, Liebman LS. Asystole during electroconvulsive therapy. J ECT. 2014;30:259–60.

16. McCully RB, Karon BL, Rummans TA, Black JL, Andreen KM, Oh JK, Seward JB, Tajik AJ. Frequency of left ventricular dysfunction after electroconvulsive therapy. Am J Cardiol. 2003;91:1147–50.
17. Hase K, Yoshioka H, Nakamura T, Kamei T, Isse K, Nakamura M. Asystole during electroconvulsive therapy. Masui. 2005;54:1268–72.
18. Wajima Z, Yoshikawa T, Ogura A, Imanaga K, Shiga T, Inoue T, Ogawa R. The effects of diltiazem on hemodynamics and seizure duration during electroconvulsive therapy. Anesth Analg. 2001;92:1327–30.
19. Wajima Z, Yoshikawa T, Ogura A, Imanaga K, Shiga T, Inoue T, Ogawa R. Intravenous verapamil blunts hyperdynamic responses during electroconvulsive therapy without altering seizure activity. Anesth Analg. 2002;95:400–2, table of contents. Erratum in: Anesth Analg 2002;95:797.
20. Wajima Z, Shiga T, Yoshikawa T, Ogura A, Inoue T, Ogawa R. Propofol alone, sevoflurane alone, and combined propofol-sevoflurane anaesthesia in electroconvulsive therapy. Anaesth Intensive Care. 2003;31:396–400.
21. Wajima Z, Shiga T, Imanaga K, Inoue T. Prophylactic continuous administration of landiolol, a novel β_1 blocker, blunts hyperdynamic responses during electroconvulsive therapy without altering seizure activity. Int J Psychiatry Clin Pract. 2010;14:132–6.
22. Simpson KH, Lynch L. Anaesthesia and electroconvulsive therapy (ECT). Anaesthesia. 1998;53:615–7.
23. Ding Z, White PF. Anesthesia for electroconvulsive therapy. Anesth Analg. 2002;94:1351–64.
24. Alpak G, Ercan S, Alici H, Bulbul F, Altunbas G, Alici D, Saricicek V, Davutoglu V. Influence of recurrent electroconvulsive therapy on cardiac function. Med Princ Pract. 2014;23:225–8.
25. Rice EH, Sombrotto LB, Markowitz JC, Leon AC. Cardiovascular morbidity in high-risk patients during ECT. Am J Psychiatry. 1994;151:1637–41.
26. Wagner KJ, Möllenberg O, Rentrop M, Werner C, Kochs EF. Guide to anaesthetic selection for electroconvulsive therapy. CNS Drugs. 2005;19:745–58.
27. Lee JT, Erbguth PH, Stevens WC, Sack RL. Modification of electroconvulsive therapy induced hypertension with nitroglycerin ointment. Anesthesiology. 1985;62:793–6.
28. Parab AL, Chaudhari LS, Apte J. Use of nitroglycerin ointment to prevent hypertensive response during electroconvulsive therapy–a study of 50 cases. J Postgrad Med. 1992;38:55–7.
29. Ciraulo D, Lind L, Salzman C, Pilon R, Elkins R. Sodium nitroprusside treatment of ECT-induced blood pressure elevations. Am J Psychiatry. 1978;135:1105–6.
30. Fu W, Stool LA, White PF, Husain MM. Is oral clonidine effective in modifying the acute hemodynamic response during electroconvulsive therapy? Anesth Analg. 1998;86:1127–30.
31. Akcaboy ZN, Akcaboy EY, Yigitbasl B, Bayam G, Dikmen B, Gogus N, Dilbaz N. Effects of remifentanil and alfentanil on seizure duration, stimulus amplitudes and recovery parameters during ECT. Acta Anaesthesiol Scand. 2005;49:1068–71.
32. Chen ST. Remifentanil: a review of its use in electroconvulsive therapy. J ECT. 2011;27:323–7.
33. Wells DG, Davies GG, Rosewarne F. Attenuation of electroconvulsive therapy induced hypertension with sublingual nifedipine. Anaesth Intensive Care. 1989;17:31–3.
34. Kalayam B, Alexopoulos GS. Nifedipene in the treatment of blood pressure rise after ECT. Convuls Ther. 1989;5:110–3.
35. Figiel GS, DeLeo B, Zorumski CF, Baker K, Goewert A, Jarvis M, Smith DS, Mattingly G, Ruwitch J. Combined use of labetalol and nifedipine in controlling the cardiovascular response from ECT. J Geriatr Psychiatry Neurol. 1993;6:20–4.
36. Avramov MN, Stool LA, White PF, Husain MM. Effects of nicardipine and labetalol on the acute hemodynamic response to electroconvulsive therapy. J Clin Anesth. 1998;10:394–400.

37. Kovac AL, Goto H, Arakawa K, Pardo MP. Esmolol bolus and infusion attenuates increases in blood pressure and heart rate during electroconvulsive therapy. Can J Anaesth. 1990;37:58–62.
38. Howie MB, Black HA, Zvara D, McSweeney TD, Martin DJ, Coffman JA. Esmolol reduces autonomic hypersensitivity and length of seizures induced by electroconvulsive therapy. Anesth Analg. 1990;71:384–8.
39. Kovac AL, Goto H, Pardo MP, Arakawa K. Comparison of two esmolol bolus doses on the haemodynamic response and seizure duration during electroconvulsive therapy. Can J Anaesth. 1991;38:204–9.
40. Weinger MB, Partridge BL, Hauger R, Mirow A. Prevention of the cardiovascular and neuroendocrine response to electroconvulsive therapy: I. Effectiveness of pretreatment regimens on hemodynamics. Anesth Analg. 1991;73:556–62.
41. Howie MB, Hiestand DC, Zvara DA, Kim PY, McSweeney TD, Coffman JA. Defining the dose range for esmolol used in electroconvulsive therapy hemodynamic attenuation. Anesth Analg. 1992;75:805–10.
42. Castelli I, Steiner LA, Kaufmann MA, Alfille PH, Schouten R, Welch CA, Drop LJ. Comparative effects of esmolol and labetalol to attenuate hyperdynamic states after electroconvulsive therapy. Anesth Analg. 1995;80:557–61.
43. van den Broek WW, Leentjens AF, Mulder PG, Kusuma A, Bruijn JA. Low-dose esmolol bolus reduces seizure duration during electroconvulsive therapy: a double-blind, placebo-controlled study. Br J Anaesth. 1999;83:271–4.
44. Foster S, Ries R. Delayed hypertension with electroconvulsive therapy. J Nerv Ment Dis. 1988;176:374–6.
45. Stoudemire A, Knos G, Gladson M, Markwalter H, Sung YF, Morris R, Cooper R. Labetalol in the control of cardiovascular responses to electroconvulsive therapy in high-risk depressed medical patients. J Clin Psychiatry. 1990;51:508–12.
46. McCall WV, Shelp FE, Weiner RD, Austin S, Harrill A. Effects of labetalol on hemodynamics and seizure duration during ECT. Convuls Ther. 1991;7:5–14.
47. American Psychiatric Association, editor. The practice of electroconvulsive therapy: recommendations for treatment, training, and priveleging, A task force report of the American Psychiatric Association. 2nd ed. Washington, DC: American Psychiatric Association; 2001. p. 136.
48. Tess AV, Smetana GW. Medical evaluation of patients undergoing electroconvulsive therapy. N Engl J Med. 2009;360:1437–44.
49. Malik MO. Fatal heart block and cardiac arrest following ECT. A case report. Br J Psychiatry. 1972;120:69–70.
50. McCall WV. Asystole in electroconvulsive therapy: report of four cases. J Clin Psychiatry. 1996;57:199–203.
51. Russ MJ, Bailine SH. Asystole and bradycardia related to anesthetic induction during ECT: a case report. J ECT. 2004;20:195–7.
52. Birkenhäger TK, Pluijms EM, Groenland TH, van den Broek WW. Severe bradycardia after anesthesia before electroconvulsive therapy. J ECT. 2010;26:53–4.
53. Dec Jr GW, Stern TA, Welch C. The effects of electroconvulsive therapy on serial electrocardiograms and serum cardiac enzyme values. A prospective study of depressed hospitalized inpatients. JAMA. 1985;253:2525–9.
54. Cockey GH, Conti CR. Electroconvulsive therapy-induced transient T-wave inversions on ECG. Clin Cardiol. 1995;18:418–20.
55. Ali PB, Tidmarsh MD. Cardiac rupture during electroconvulsive therapy. Anaesthesia. 1997;52:884–6.
56. Lopez-Gomez D, Sanchez-Corral MA, Cobo JV, Jara F, Esplugas E. Myocardial infarction after electroconvulsive therapy. Rev Esp Cardiol. 1999;52:536.

57. Messina AG, Paranicas M, Katz B, Markowitz J, Yao FS, Devereux RB. Effect of electroconvulsive therapy on the electrocardiogram and echocardiogram. Anesth Analg. 1992;75:511–4.
58. Go O, Mukherjee R, Bhatta L, Carhart Jr R, Villarreal D. Myocardial stunning after electroconvulsive therapy in patients with an apparently normal heart. J ECT. 2009;25:117–20.
59. Satterthwaite TD, Cristancho MA, Alici Y, Weiss D, O'Reardon JP. Electroconvulsive therapy in a 72-year-old woman with a history of Takotsubo cardiomyopathy: a case report and review of the literature. Brain Stimul. 2009;2:238–40.
60. Beach SR, Wichman CL, Canterbury RJ. Takotsubo cardiomyopathy after electroconvulsive therapy. Psychosomatics. 2010;51:432–6.
61. Celano CM, Torri A, Seiner S. Takotsubo cardiomyopathy after electroconvulsive therapy: a case report and review. J ECT. 2011;27:221–3.
62. Narayanan A, Russell MD, Sundararaman S, Shankar KK, Artman B. Takotsubo cardiomyopathy following electroconvulsive therapy: an increasingly recognised phenomenon. BMJ Case Rep. 2014;2014.
63. Sharkey SW, Lesser JR, Zenovich AG, Maron MS, Lindberg J, Longe TF, Maron BJ. Acute and reversible cardiomyopathy provoked by stress in women from the United States. Circulation. 2005;111:472–9.
64. Kokras N, Politis AM, Zervas IM, Pappa D, Markatou M, Katirtzoglou E, Papadimitriou GN. Cardiac rhythm management devices and electroconvulsive therapy: a critical review apropos of a depressed patient with a pacemaker. J ECT. 2011;27:214–20.
65. Gosselink MJ, Schenkeveld KW, Trines SA, van Vliet IM. Successful electroconvulsive therapy in a 95-year-old man with a cardiac pacemaker–a case report. Am J Geriatr Psychiatry. 2011;19:678–9.
66. Dolenc TJ, Barnes RD, Hayes DL, Rasmussen KG. Electroconvulsive therapy in patients with cardiac pacemakers and implantable cardioverter defibrillators. Pacing Clin Electrophysiol. 2004;27:1257–63.
67. Zavorotnyy M, Zwanzger P. Prolonged apnea during electroconvulsive therapy in monozygotic twins: case reports. Ann Gen Psychiatry. 2011;10:30.
68. Naguib M, Lien CA. Pharmacology of muscle relaxant and their antagonists. In: Miller RD, editor. Miller's anesthesia, vol. 1. 7th ed. Philadelphia: Churchill Livingstone Elsevier; 2010. p. 859–911.
69. Packman PM, Meyer DA, Verdun RM. Hazards of succinylcholine administration during electrotherapy. Arch Gen Psychiatry. 1978;35:1137–41.
70. De Hert M, Einfinger G, Scherpenberg E, Wampers M, Peuskens J. The prevention of deep venous thrombosis in physically restrained patients with schizophrenia. Int J Clin Pract. 2010;64:1109–15.
71. Medda P, Fornaro M, Fratta S, Callari A, Manzo V, Ciaponi B, Perugi G. A case of deep venous thrombosis following protracted catatonic immobility recovered with electroconvulsive therapy: the relevance for an early intervention. Gen Hosp Psychiatry. 2012;34:209.e5–7.
72. Clinebell K, Azzam PN, Gopalan P, Haskett R. Guidelines for preventing common medical complications of catatonia: case report and literature review. J Clin Psychiatry. 2014;75:644–51.
73. Weber DL, Ruvolo C, Cashin P. Sudden death following electroconvulsive therapy. N Y State J Med. 1973;73:1000–1.
74. Mamah D, Lammle M, Isenberg KE. Pulmonary embolism after ECT. J ECT. 2005;21:39–40.
75. Suzuki K, Takamatsu K, Takano T, Tanabe Y, Fujiyama K, Matsuoka H. Safety of electroconvulsive therapy in psychiatric patients shortly after the occurrence of pulmonary embolism. J ECT. 2008;24:286–8.

76. Singh G, Wahi S. Pulmonary embolism in the ECT patient: a case report and discussion. Gen Hosp Psychiatry. 2008;30:87–9.
77. Kalava A, Kalstein A, Koyfman S, Mardakh S, Yarmush JM, Schianodicola J. Pulseless electrical activity during electroconvulsive therapy: a case report. BMC Anesthesiol. 2012;12:8.
78. Kurnutala LN, Kamath S, Koyfman S, Yarmush J, SchianodiCola J. Aspiration during electroconvulsive therapy under general anesthesia. J ECT. 2013;29, e68.
79. Zibrak JD, Jensen WA, Bloomingdale K. Aspiration pneumonitis following electroconvulsive therapy in patients with gastroparesis. Biol Psychiatry. 1988;24:812–4.
80. Abrams R. Technique of electoconvulsive therapy: theory. In: Abrams R, editor. Electroconvulsive therapy. 4th ed. New York: Oxford University Press; 2002. p. 168.
81. Tecoult E, Nathan N. Morbidity in electroconvulsive therapy. Eur J Anaesthesiol. 2001;18:511–8.
82. Swartz CM. Electroconvulsive therapy emergence agitation and succinylcholine dose. J Nerv Ment Dis. 1990;178:455–7.
83. Meignan ML. Morbidity in electroconvulsive therapy. Eur J Anaesthesiol. 2002;19:614–5; author reply 5.
84. Wild B, Eschweiler GW, Bartels M. Morbidity in electroconvulsive therapy. Eur J Anaesthesiol. 2002;19:616.
85. Hasler WL. Gastroparesis. Curr Opin Gastroenterol. 2012;28:621–8.
86. American Society of Anesthesiologists Committee. Practice guidelines for preoperative fasting and the use of pharmacologic agents to reduce the risk of pulmonary aspiration: application to healthy patients undergoing elective procedures: an updated report by the American Society of Anesthesiologists Committee on Standards and Practice Parameters. Anesthesiology. 2011;114:495–511.
87. Hagberg CA, Artime CA. Airway mangement in the adult. In: Miller RD, editor. Miller's anesthesia, vol. 1. 8th ed. Philadelphia: Elsevier Saunders; 2015. p. 1647–83.
88. Smith I, Kranke P, Murat I, Smith A, O'Sullivan G, Soreide E, Spies C, in't Veld B. Perioperative fasting in adults and children: guidelines from the European Society of Anaesthesiology. Eur J Anaesthesiol. 2011;28:556–69.
89. Berrios GE, Sage G. Patients who break their fast before ECT. Br J Psychiatry. 1986;149:294–5.
90. Buisseret P. Acute pulmonary oedema following grand mal epilepsy and as a complication of electric shock therapy. Br J Dis Chest. 1982;76:194–5.
91. Cochran M, DeBattista C, Schmiesing C, Brock-Utne JG. Negative-pressure pulmonary edema: a potential hazard in patients undergoing ECT. J ECT. 1999;15:168–70.
92. Hatta K, Kitajima A, Ito M, Usui C, Arai H. Pulmonary edema after electroconvulsive therapy in a patient treated for long-standing asthma with a β_2 stimulant. J ECT. 2007;23:26–7.
93. Myers CL, Gopalka A, Glick D, Goldman MB, Dinwiddie SH. A case of negative-pressure pulmonary edema after electroconvulsive therapy. J ECT. 2007;23:281–3.
94. Ring BS, Parnass SM, Shulman RB, Phelan J, Khan SA. Cardiogenic shock after electroconvulsive therapy. Anesthesiology. 1996;84:1511–3.
95. Wayne SL, O'Donovan CA, McCall WV, Link K. Postictal neurogenic pulmonary edema: experience from an ECT model. Convuls Ther. 1997;13:181–4.
96. Tsutsumi N, Tohdoh Y, Kawana S, Kozuka Y, Namiki A. A case of pulmonary edema after electroconvulsive therapy under propofol anesthesia. Masui. 2001;50:525–7.
97. Price JW, Price JR, Perry TL. Excessive hypertension and pulmonary edema after electroconvulsive therapy. J ECT. 2005;21:174–7.
98. Graham Jr JM, Tackels D, Dibbern K, Superneau D, Rogers C, Corning K, Schwartz CE. FG syndrome: report of three new families with linkage to Xq12-q22.1. Am J Med Genet. 1998;80:145–56.

99. Salmo EN, Connolly CE. Mortality in epilepsy in the west of Ireland: a 10-year review. Ir J Med Sci. 2002;171:199–201.
100. Reynolds RW. Pulmonary edema as a consequence of hypothalamic lesions in rats. Science. 1963;141:930–2.
101. Sarnoff SJ, Sarnoff LC. Neurohemodynamics of pulmonary edema. II. The role of sympathetic pathways in the elevation of pulmonary and stemic vascular pressures following the intracisternal injection of fibrin. Circulation. 1952;6:51–62.
102. Brashear RE, Pamintuan RL. Increased pulmonary diffusing capacity and elevated cerebrospinal fluid pressure. J Appl Physiol. 1971;30:844–6.
103. Sarnoff SJ, Berglund E. Neurohemodynamics of pulmonary edema. IV. Effect of systemic vasoconstriction and subsequent vasodilation on flow and pressures in systemic and pulmonary vascular beds. Am J Physiol. 1952;170:588–600.
104. Robin ED, Cross CE, Zelis R. Pulmonary edema. 1. N Engl J Med. 1973;288:239–46.
105. Gandhi SK, Powers JC, Nomeir AM, Fowle K, Kitzman DW, Rankin KM, Little WC. The pathogenesis of acute pulmonary edema associated with hypertension. N Engl J Med. 2001;344:17–22.
106. Fawver J, Milstein V. Asthma/emphysema complication of electroconvulsive therapy: a case study. Convuls Ther. 1985;1:61–4.
107. Kurup V. Respiratory diseases. In: Hines RL, Marschall KE, editors. Stoelting's ansthesia and co-existing disease. 5th ed. Philadelphia: Saunders Elsevier; 2008. p. 161–97.
108. National Asthma Education and Prevention Program. Expert Panel Report 3 (EPR-3): guidelines for the diagnosis and management of Asthma-Summary Report 2007. J Allergy Clin Immunol. 2007;120:S94–138.
109. Lougheed MD, Leniere C, Ducharme FM, Licskai C, Dell SD, Rowe BH, FitzGerald M, Leigh R, Watson W, Boulet LP. Canadian Thoracic Society 2012 guideline update: diagnosis and management of asthma in preschoolers, children and adults: executive summary. Can Respir J. 2012;19:e81–8.
110. Vestbo J, Hurd SS, Agusti AG, Jones PW, Vogelmeier C, Anzueto A, Barnes PJ, Fabbri LM, Martinez FJ, Nishimura M, Stockley RA, Sin DD, Rodriguez-Roisin R. Global strategy for the diagnosis, management, and prevention of chronic obstructive pulmonary disease: GOLD executive summary. Am J Respir Crit Care Med. 2013;187:347–65.
111. Nagele P, Hüpfl M. Anesthesia and prehospital emergency and trauma care. In: Miller RD, editor. Miller's anesthesia, vol. 2. 8th ed. Philadelphia: Elsevier Saunders; 2015. p. 2460–78.
112. Krystal AD. Managing the ECT seizure. In: Mankad MV, Beyer JL, Weiner RD, Krystal AD, editors. Clinical manual of electroconvulsive therapy. Arlington: American Psychiatric Publishing, Inc.; 2010. p. 149–57.
113. Weiner RD, Coffey CE, Krystal AD. The monitoring and management of electrically induced seizures. Psychiatr Clin North Am. 1991;14:845–69.
114. American Psychiatric Association. The practice of electroconvulsive therapy: recommendations for treatment, training, and priveleging, A task force report of the American Psychiatric Association. 2nd ed. Washington, DC: American Psychiatric Association; 2001. p. 193–4.
115. Walter G, Rey JM. An epidemiological study of the use of ECT in adolescents. J Am Acad Child Adolesc Psychiatry. 1997;36:809–15.
116. American Psychiatric Association, editor. The practice of electroconvulsive therapy: recommendations for treatment, training, and priveleging, A task force report of the American Psychiatric Association. 2nd ed. Washington, DC: American Psychiatric Association; 2001. p. 77–95.
117. Saito S, Miyoshi S, Yoshikawa D, Shimada H, Morita T, Kitani Y. Regional cerebral oxygen saturation during electroconvulsive therapy: monitoring by near-infrared spectrophotometry. Anesth Analg. 1996;83:726–30.
118. Pansare NH, Trenton AJ, Pelchat R. Electroconvulsive therapy performed 6 days after repair of an intracranial aneurysm using a liquid embolic system. J ECT. 2014;30:e19–21.

119. Maltbie AA, Wingfield MS, Volow MR, Weiner RD, Sullivan JL, Cavenar Jr JO. Electroconvulsive therapy in the presence of brain tumor. Case reports and an evaluation of risk. J Nerv Ment Dis. 1980;168:400–5.
120. Rasmussen KG, Perry CL, Sutor B, Moore KM. ECT in patients with intracranial masses. J Neuropsychiatry Clin Neurosci. 2007;19:191–3.
121. Patkar AA, Hill KP, Weinstein SP, Schwartz SL. ECT in the presence of brain tumor and increased intracranial pressure: evaluation and reduction of risk. J ECT. 2000;16:189–97.
122. Kramer BA. Use of ECT in California, 1977–1983. Am J Psychiatry. 1985;142:1190–2.
123. Najjar F, Guttmacher LB. ECT in the presence of intracranial aneurysm. J ECT. 1998;14:266–71.
124. Martin M, Figiel G, Mattingly G, Zorumski CF, Jarvis MR. ECT-induced interictal delirium in patients with a history of a CVA. J Geriatr Psychiatry Neurol. 1992;5:149–55.
125. Selim M. Perioperative stroke. N Engl J Med. 2007;356:706–13.
126. Awasthy N, Chand K. Subdural hematoma – a complication of electro convulsive therapy. Pak J Med Sci. 2005;21:491–3.
127. Saha D, Bisui B, Thakurta RG, Ghoshmaulik S, Singh OP. Chronic subdural hematoma following electro convulsive therapy. Indian J Psychol Med. 2012;34:181–3.
128. Kulkarni RR, Melkundi S. Subdural hematoma: an adverse event of electroconvulsive therapy-case report and literature review. Case Rep Psychiatry. 2012;2012:585303.
129. Dinwiddie SH, Huo D, Gottlieb O. The course of myalgia and headache after electroconvulsive therapy. J ECT. 2010;26:116–20.
130. Kertesz DP, Trabekin O, Vanetik MS. Headache treatment after electroconvulsive treatment: a single-blinded trial comparator between Eletriptan and Paracetamol. J ECT. 2015;31:105–9.
131. Leung M, Hollander Y, Brown GR. Pretreatment with ibuprofen to prevent electroconvulsive therapy-induced headache. J Clin Psychiatry. 2003;64:551–3.
132. Markowitz JS, Kellner CH, DeVane CL, Beale MD, Folk J, Burns C, Liston HL. Intranasal sumatriptan in post-ECT headache: results of an open-label trial. J ECT. 2001;17:280–3.
133. Kellner CH, Bryson EO. Electroconvulsive therapy anesthesia technique: minimalist versus maximally managed. J ECT. 2013;29:153–5.
134. DeBattista C, Mueller K. Sumatriptan prophylaxis for postelectroconvulsive therapy headaches. Headache. 1995;35:502–3.
135. Yatham LN, Liddle PF, Lam RW, Zis AP, Stoessl AJ, Sossi V, Adam MJ, Ruth TJ. Effect of electroconvulsive therapy on brain 5-HT_2 receptors in major depression. Br J Psychiatry. 2010;196:474–9.
136. Mirzakhani H, Welch CA, Eikermann M, Nozari A. Neuromuscular blocking agents for electroconvulsive therapy: a systematic review. Acta Anaesthesiol Scand. 2012;56:3–16.
137. Murphy GS, De Boer HD, Eriksson LI, Miller RD. Reversal (antagonism) of neuromuscular blockade. In: Miller RD, editor. Miller's anesthesia, vol. 1. 8th ed. Philadelphia: Elsevier Saunders; 2015. p. 995–1027.
138. Jain M, Arya A, Jha DK, Mehrotra S, Sarma U, Mehra A. Aggravated spinal cord compression following electroconvulsive therapy. J Anaesthesiol Clin Pharmacol. 2010;26:572.
139. Briggs MC, Popeo DM, Pasculli RM, Bryson EO, Kellner CH. Safe resumption of electroconvulsive therapy (ECT) after vertebroplasty. Int J Geriatr Psychiatry. 2012;27:984–5.
140. Kellner CH, Tolhurst JE, Burns CM. ECT in the presence of severe cervical spine disease. Convuls Ther. 1991;7:52–5.
141. O'Connell RA. A review of the use of electroconvulsive therapy. Hosp Community Psychiatry. 1982;33:469–73.
142. Shaheen MA, Sabet NA. Bilateral simultaneous fracture of the femoral neck following electrical shock. Injury. 1984;16:13–4.
143. Nott MR, Watts JS. A fractured hip during electro-convulsive therapy. Eur J Anaesthesiol. 1999;16:265–7.

144. Browne AO, Sheehan JM. Bilateral central dislocation of the hip: a case report. Orthop Rev. 1986;15:733–5.
145. Ribbans WJ. Bilateral anterior dislocation of the shoulder following a grand-mal convulsion. Br J Clin Pract. 1989;43:181–2.
146. Rodia F, Ventura A, Touloupakis G, Theodorakis E, Ceretti M. Missed posterior shoulder dislocation and McLaughlin lesion after an electrocution accident. Chin J Traumatol. 2012;15:376–8.
147. Rawat S, Meena S, Gangari SK, Lohia LK. Anterior dislocation of shoulder in eclampsia: a case report. Chin J Traumatol. 2012;15:249–50.
148. Auriacombe M, Reneric JP, Usandizaga D, Gomez F, Combourieu I, Tignol J. Post-ECT agitation and plasma lactate concentrations. J ECT. 2000;16:263–7.
149. Fink M. Post-ECT Delirium. Convuls Ther. 1993;9:326–30.
150. Augoustides JG, Greenblatt E, Abbas MA, O'Reardon JP, Datto CJ. Clinical approach to agitation after electroconvulsive therapy: a case report and literature review. J ECT. 2002;18:213–7.
151. Cohen MB, Stewart JT. Treatment of post-electroconvulsive therapy agitation with dexmedetomidine. J ECT. 2013;29:e23–4.
152. Aneja J, Grover S, Agarwal M, Kaushik S. Use of electroconvulsive therapy in the presence of glaucoma: a case report and review of literature. Indian J Psychol Med. 2013;35:80–3.
153. Good MS, Dolenc TJ, Rasmussen KG. Electroconvulsive therapy in a patient with glaucoma. J ECT. 2004;20:48–9.
154. Boroojeny SB, Tabatabai NH, Babakhani B, Babakhani S, Moody Z. The effect of electroconvulsive therapy using propofol and succinylcholine on the intraocular pressure. Middle East J Anesthesiol. 2012;21:713–7.
155. Sibony PA. ECT risks in glaucoma. Convuls Ther. 1985;1:283–5.
156. American Psychiatric Association. The practice of electroconvulsive therapy: recommendations for treatment, training, and priveleging, A task force report of the American Psychiatric Association. 2nd ed. Washington, DC: American Psychiatric Association; 2001. p. 41–2.
157. Waters DJ, Mapleson WW. Suxamethonium pains: hypothesis and observation. Anaesthesia. 1971;26:127–41.
158. McLoughlin C, Elliott P, McCarthy G, Mirakhur RK. Muscle pains and biochemical changes following suxamethonium administration after six pretreatment regimens. Anaesthesia. 1992;47:202–6.
159. Rasmussen KG, Petersen KN, Sticka JL, Wieme LJ, Zosel JH, Marienau ME, Ryan DA, Schroeder DR, Stevens SR, Hooten WM, Spackman TN. Correlates of myalgia in electroconvulsive therapy. J ECT. 2008;24:84–7.
160. Morris AJ, Roche SA, Bentham P, Wright J. A dental risk management protocol for electroconvulsive therapy. J ECT. 2002;18:84–9.
161. Kiran S, Bala R, Singh T. Dental protection during modified electroconvulsive therapy using roll-gauze mouth gag. J ECT. 2009;25:74–5.
162. McClure RE. A device for preventing dental injuries during ECT. Hosp Commun Psychiatry. 1969;20:357–9.
163. McCall WV, Minneman SA, Minneman SA, Weiner RD, Shelp FE, Austin S. Dental pathology in ECT patients prior to treatment. Convuls Ther. 1992;8:19–24.
164. American Psychiatric Association. The practice of electroconvulsive therapy: recommendations for treatment, training, and priveleging, A task force report of the American Psychiatric Association. 2nd ed. Washington, DC: American Psychiatric Association; 2001. p. 64–5.
165. Li TC, Shiah IS, Sun CJ, Tzang RF, Huang KC, Lee WK. Mirtazapine relieves post-electroconvulsive therapy headaches and nausea: a case series and review of the literature. J ECT. 2011;27:165–7.
166. Kramer BA. Anticholinergics and ECT. Convuls Ther. 1993;9:293–300.

167. Kellner CH, Li D, Maron L. Anesthesia for electroconvulsive therapy. In: Swartz CM, editor. Electroconvulsive and neuromodulation therapies. New York: Cambridge University Press; 2009. p. 414–5.
168. Greenan J, Dewar M, Jones CJ. Intravenous glycopyrrolate and atropine at induction of anaesthesia: a comparison. J R Soc Med. 1983;76:369–71.
169. Manjunatha N, Ram Kumar GS, Vidyendaran R, Muralidharan K, John JP. Delayed onset, protracted delirium and aspiration pneumonitis associated with a combination of clozapine and electroconvulsive therapy. Indian J Psychol Med. 2011;33:80–2.
170. Reddy S, Nobler MS. Dangerous hyperglycemia associated with electroconvulsive therapy. Convuls Ther. 1996;12:99–103.
171. Shimabukuro D, Liu LL. Cardiopulmonary resuscitation. In: Miller RD, Pardo Jr MC, editors. Basics of anesthesia. 6th ed. Philadelphia: Elsevier Saunders; 2011. p. 727.
172. Vervloet D, Magnan A, Birnbaum J, Pradal M. Allergic emergencies seen in surgical suites. Clin Rev Allergy Immunol. 1999;17:459–67.
173. Laxenaire MC. Epidemiology of anesthetic anaphylactoid reactions. Fourth multicenter survey (July 1994-December 1996). Ann Fr Anesth Reanim. 1999;18:796–809.
174. Hepner DL, Castells MC. Anaphylaxis during the perioperative period. Anesth Analg. 2003;97:1381–95.
175. Ebo DG, Fisher MM, Hagendorens MM, Bridts CH, Stevens WJ. Anaphylaxis during anaesthesia: diagnostic approach. Allergy. 2007;62:471–87.
176. Fisher MM, Baldo BA. The incidence and clinical features of anaphylactic reactions during anesthesia in Australia. Ann Fr Anesth Reanim. 1993;12:97–104.
177. Fasting S, Gisvold SE. Serious intraoperative problems–a five-year review of 83,844 anesthetics. Can J Anaesth. 2002;49:545–53.
178. Mertes PM, Laxenaire MC, Alla F. Anaphylactic and anaphylactoid reactions occurring during anesthesia in France in 1999–2000. Anesthesiology. 2003;99:536–45.
179. Sadleir PH, Clarke RC, Bunning DL, Platt PR. Anaphylaxis to neuromuscular blocking drugs: incidence and cross-reactivity in Western Australia from 2002 to 2011. Br J Anaesth. 2013;110:981–7.
180. Reddy JI, Cooke PJ, van Schalkwyk JM, Hannam JA, Fitzharris P, Mitchell SJ. Anaphylaxis is more common with rocuronium and succinylcholine than with atracurium. Anesthesiology. 2015;122:39–45.
181. Currie M, Webb RK, Williamson JA, Russell WJ, Mackay P, The Australian Incident Monitoring Study. Clinical anaphylaxis: an analysis of 2000 incident reports. Anaesth Intensive Care. 1993;21:621–5.
182. Mertes PM, Aimone-Gastin I, Gueant-Rodriguez RM, Mouton-Faivre C, Audibert G, O'Brien J, Frendt D, Brezeanu M, Bouaziz H, Gueant JL. Hypersensitivity reactions to neuromuscular blocking agents. Curr Pharm Des. 2008;14:2809–25.
183. Mitsuhata H, Matsumoto S, Hasegawa J. The epidemiology and clinical features of anaphylactic and anaphylactoid reactions in the perioperative period in Japan. Masui. 1992;41:1664–9.
184. Axon AD, Hunter JM. Editorial III: Anaphylaxis and anaesthesia–all clear now? Br J Anaesth. 2004;93:501–4.
185. Misra UK, Kalita J, Vajpeyee A, Mandhani A, Sharma RK. Bladder rupture: a rare complication of tonic-clonic seizures. QJM. 2003;96:542–3.
186. Irving AD, Drayson AM. Bladder rupture during ECT. Br J Psychiatry. 1984;144:670.
187. O'Brien PD, Morgan DH. Bladder rupture during ECT. Convuls Ther. 1991;7:56–9.
188. Abrams R. Technique of electoconvulsive therapy: theory. In: Abrams R, editor. Electroconvulsive therapy. 4th ed. New York: Oxford University Press; 2002. p. 168–9.
189. van Schaik AM, Klumpers UM, de Gast HM, Kubbe DA, Stek ML. Gastric rupture after electroconvulsive therapy. J ECT. 2006;22:153–4.
190. Devanand DP, Prudic J, Sackeim HA. Electroconvulsive therapy-induced hypomania is uncommon. Convuls Ther. 1992;8:296–8.

191. American Psychiatric Association. The practice of electroconvulsive therapy: recommendations for treatment, training, and priveleging, A task force report of the American Psychiatric Association. 2nd ed. Washington, DC: American Psychiatric Association; 2001. p. 66–73.
192. UK ECT Review Group. Efficacy and safety of electroconvulsive therapy in depressive disorders: a systematic review and meta-analysis. Lancet. 2003;361:799–808.
193. Sackeim HA, Prudic J, Fuller R, Keilp J, Lavori PW, Olfson M. The cognitive effects of electroconvulsive therapy in community settings. Neuropsychopharmacology. 2007;32:244–54.
194. Rose D, Fleischmann P, Wykes T, Leese M, Bindman J. Patients' perspectives on electroconvulsive therapy: systematic review. BMJ. 2003;326:1363.